Five Element Acupuncture

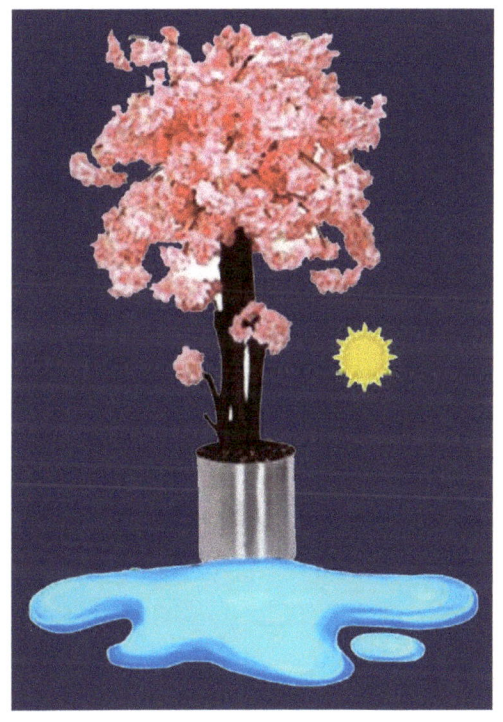

DR. ADNAN UZUN

August, 2024

İSTANBUL

Book Name: *FIVE ELEMENT ACUPUNCTURE*
Author: Op. Dr. Adnan Uzun
Editorial & Cover: © E-Kitap Projesi
Publisher: E-Kitap Projesi & Cheapest Books

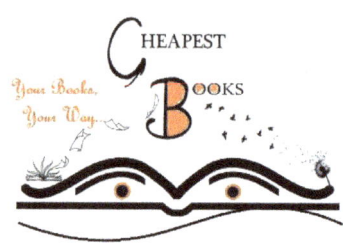

www.cheapestboooks.com
www.ekitaprojesi.com
Publisher Certificate No: 45502
İstanbul, August / 2024
ISBN: 978-625-6235-14-4
eISBN: 978-625-6235-13-7

Contact
E-Mail:
drauzun@hotmail.com

For reply and your comments:
www.ekitaprojesi.com/books/five-element-acupuncture
www.facebook.com/EKitapProjesi

© **Dr. Adnan Uzun, 2024**
Printing and publication rights belong to the author. Without his permission no part can be reproduced or republished.

Table of Contents:

AUTOBİOGRAPHY 6
PREFACE 8
DEFINITION OF ACUPUNCTURE 10
DEFINITION OF THE FIVE ELEMENT THEORY 15
HISTORY OF THE FIVE ELEMENT THEORY..................18
INTRODUCTION TO FIVE ELEMENT THEORY 20
THE FIVE ELEMENTS AND THE CONCEPTS RELATED
TO THEM 22
   ORGANS..25
   SENSE ORGANS..27
   FEELINGS...28
   SEASONS AND ENVIRONMENTAL FACTORS...........30
   FLAVORS..32
   COLORS 33
   SOUNDS 34
   SOULS 34
      PO (CORPORAL SOUL) 35
      SHEN..36
      HUN (ETHERIC SOUL) 38
      ZHI...42
      Yİ (İNTELLECT)..42
   SMELL...43
   MUSIC AND SHEET NOTES.......................................44
   GRAİNS 46
   DIRECTIONS AND NUMBERS 47
MUTUAL RELATIONSHIPS OF THE FIVE ELEMENTS....49
   1. MOTHER-SON INTERACTION (SHENG CYCLE).....50
   2. CONTROLLER INTERACTION (KE CYCLE)............54
   3. EXCESSIVE SUPPRESSİVE INTERACTION...........56
   4. İNSULTİNG INTERACTION......................................57
CRITICAL APPROACHES TO THE FIVE ELEMENTS
THEORY 61

FIRST CRITICISM:	61
ANSWER TO THE FIRST CRITICISM:	62
SECOND CRITICISM:	63
ANSWER TO THE SECOND CRITICISM:	64
ENERGY VİEWS OF SISTER ORGANS AND THEIR RELATED MERIDIANS	67
TERMINOLOGICAL INFORMATION	73
THREE STEPS TO APPROACHING DISEASES	74
FIRST STEP	77
FIND THE FAULTY POOL	77
SECOND STEP	96
CHECK THE TEMPERATURE OF THE POOL	96
THİRD STEP	133
EDIT THE TEMPERATURE OF THE FAULTY POOL	133
FIVE ELEMENT ACUPUNCTURE	145
FIVE SHU POINTS OF THE LUNG MERIDIAN	151
FIVE SHU POINTS OF THE LARGE INTESTINE MERIDIAN	157
SAMPLE CASES ABOUT THE METAL ELEMENT	161
EXAMPLE CASE 1 (ACUTE SINUSITIS):	161
EXAMPLE CASE 2 (FREQUENTLY RECURRENT UPPER RESPIRATORY TRACT INFECTION):	163
EXAMPLE CASE 3 (ASTHMA AND CHRONIC CONSTIPATION)	166
EXAMPLE CASE 4 (ULCERATIVE COLITIS AND ASTHMA):	168
EXAMPLE CASE 5 (SHOULDER PAIN):	171
EXAMPLE CASE 6 (LATERAL EPICONDYLITIS):	174
STOMACH MERIDIAN FIVE SHU POINTS	176
FIVE SHU POINTS OF THE SPLEEN MERIDIAN	178
SAMPLE CASES RELATED TO EARTH ELEMENT	181
EXAMPLE CASE 1 (CHRONIC GASTRITIS):	181
EXAMPLE CASE 2 (LYMPHEDEMA):	183
EXAMPLE CASE 3 (REPEAT ANKLE SPRAIN):	185
EXAMPLE CASE 4 (ACUTE TONSILLITIS):	186
HEART MERIDIAN FIVE SHU POINTS	191

FIVE SHU POINTS OF THE SMALL INTESTINE MERIDIAN 195
PERICHARD MERIDIAN FIVE SHU POINTS 198
SANJIAO MERIDIAN FIVE SHU POINTS 201
CASE STUDIES RELATED TO THE ELEMENT FIRE.....204
   EXAMPLE CASE 1 (ANGINA PECTORIS):..................204
   EXAMPLE CASE 2 (ILEUS IN THE SMALL INTESTINE): 206
   EXAMPLE CASE 3 (PAINFUL AFT ON TONGUE): 210
   EXAMPLE CASE 4 (HYPERTENSION):........................213
   EXAMPLE CASE 5 (CARPAL TUNNEL SYNDROME): 216
   EXAMPLE CASE 6 (STUTTERING): 219
FIVE SHU POINTS OF THE LIVER MERIDIAN 221
GALLBLADDER MERIDIAN FIVE SHU POINTS 224
SAMPLE CASES ABOUT THE WOOD ELEMENT 228
   EXAMPLE CASE 1 (MIGRINE):.....................................228
   EXAMPLE CASE 2 (ACUTE CHOLECYSTITIS): 233
   EXAMPLE CASE 3 (EPILEPSY):...................................236
   EXAMPLE CASE 4 (VERTIGO): 240
   EXAMPLE CASE 5 (VERTIGO AND WAIST PAIN): 246
   EXAMPLE CASE 6 (MIGRAINE AND ANKLE TENDON RUPTURE) 249
KIDNEY MERIDIAN FIVE SHU POINTS 254
BLADDER MERIDIAN FIVE SHU POINTS......................256
SAMPLE CASES ABOUT THE WATER ELEMENT.........260
   EXAMPLE CASE1 (BACK PAIN): 260
   EXAMPLE CASE 2 (HEARING LOSS): 265
   EXAMPLE CASE 3 (ACCHILLES TENDENITIS): 269
   EXAMPLE CASE 4 (COMMON JOINT PAIN): 273
   EXAMPLE CASE 5 (TINNITUS): 275
RESOURCES..280

AUTOBİOGRAPHY

I was born in Samsun Çarşamba in 1977. I completed my primary, secondary and high school education in Çarşamba. I was accepted to Cerrahpaşa Faculty of Medicine in 1995 and graduated in 2001. I completed my ENT specialization at Ankara Numune Education and Research Hospital. Between 2001 and 2015, I worked at Kaman State Hospital, Ardahan State Hospital and various private hospitals in Ankara. In 2015-2016, I became interested in Traditional Chinese Medicine and started researching and reading in this direction. Traditional Chinese Medicine is a medical system that includes many treatment options. Since acupuncture treatment is the most important of these options and Traditional Chinese Medicine education in our country is mainly given through acupuncture, I focused my research more in this direction. The fact that most of the resources about acupuncture are in English and that I do not know English well enough was my biggest obstacle. My interest in acupuncture helped me learn enough English to understand what I was reading. As I read, I saw that acupuncture did not have a standard application method and that there were many different schools in different parts of the world. I had embarked on such a path that my interest and love for acupuncture had reached a level I could not describe. I decided to continue the education process by getting a certificate. In 2017, I attended the certified course opened by Yıldırım Beyazıt University and completed my education. Of course, acupuncture training is not a branch of science that you can say "it's over now". I believe that the best way to learn is to share what you have learned with others. This belief led me to write two books in 2019, "Systematic Acupuncture" and "Ear Acupuncture". Theoretical knowledge that is not put into practice is doomed to be forgotten. During this process, I wanted to put my knowledge into practice and write a new book that would be easily understood by everyone in the light of the experiences I gained. I am currently practicing my profession in a private medical center. I am married and have two children.

Op. Dr. Adnan Uzun

PREFACE

Praise be to God, and blessings be upon his Messenger, who gave me the opportunity to finish this book called "Five element acupuncture" after the books "Systematic acupuncture" and "Ear acupuncture" and present it to you, the reader. Acupuncture is a part of TCM and requires looking at the person from a holistic perspective. Acupuncture education and training is a very enjoyable process. It requires a long marathon. Unfortunately, I have witnessed many physician friends who did not use the correct method in this marathon, abandoning this race. I frequently used the art of simile in the approach in this book, where we explain acupuncture through a sequence of logic. Thus, abstract subjects and concepts that were difficult to understand by friends trained in Western Medicine became much easier to understand. If the reader learns this science in line with the principles I have explained, he will be able to make his own prescription for all kinds of diseases and will avoid being a point acupuncturist.

In the book, I touched upon the basic acupuncture information that I deemed necessary regarding my subject, and tried to give the message I wanted to give directly, without extending the subject too much. I drew a picture for you in the book. I did not draw the whole picture, but the parts that I deemed important. I went into detail on some pieces that serve as touchstones to understand the whole picture. Thus, when the reader fully understands the cornerstone parts of the picture, he will be able to fill in the gaps in the picture very easily. This style of narration enabled us to convey, in a short content, a subject that could only be understood if volumes of books were written. Therefore, do not be fooled by the small volume of the book. The knowledge you will gain from many reference books that explain the subject in detail will not be more than the knowledge you will gain from this book.

The book was written with an English translation. This book, in which acupuncture enthusiasts will find answers to many issues that they cannot understand, will fill a huge gap in its field with the explanations it provides on many issues whose boundaries are not clear.

Op. Dr. Adnan Uzun

DEFINITION OF ACUPUNCTURE

According to TCM, each organ has its own energy channel called meridian. When the energy flow in these meridians is interrupted for any reason, meridian-related or organ-related symptoms may occur. Let's expand this sentence a little by looking at the course of the lung meridian. The lung meridian starts from the thorax, passes through the shoulder, arm, elbow and wrist and ends at the thumb (Figure-1). When there is a blockage in energy along the course of the meridian, musculoskeletal diseases such as shoulder pain, elbow pain, wrist pain or finger pain may occur. Or, if pain does not occur, it may be reflected clinically in the form of skin paresthesia or skin rashes along the course of the meridian. The disease may not be reflected in the clinic due to problems related to the meridian course. It may also occur with organ-related symptoms. If we continue with the lung example, the patient may present with organ-related symptoms such as cough, hoarseness, and shortness of breath.

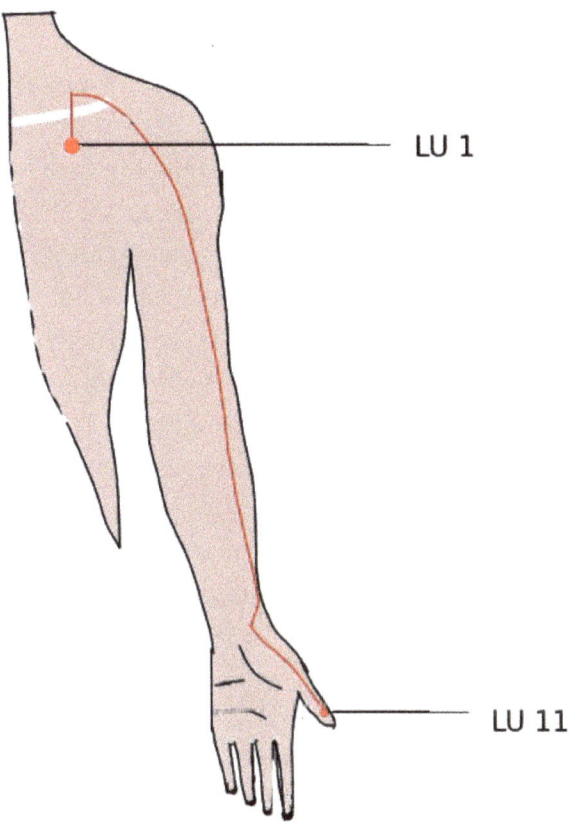

Figure 1: Lung meridian course

According to the five element theory, each organ has associated sensory organs, emotions and tissues. The patient may also come to the clinic with complaints related to these. To understand this sentence better, see Figure 2. You see the kidney tree in the figure. As we will see later, according to TCM, every organ has a sister organ. The sister organ of the kidney is the bladder. Therefore, think of this tree with its sister as the kidney and bladder tree, which according to the five element theory, these two organs are represented by the water element. When there is any energy imbalance in the water element, it may come to us with symptoms such as heel pain, knee pain, lower back pain along the meridian course. The sensory organ associated with the water element is the ear. For this reason, the patient may apply to us with complaints such as decreased hearing or buzzing and ringing in the ears. There are many tissues associated with the water element. These are bones, hair, teeth, neural tissues and small joints. Therefore, the patient may come to us with toothache, widespread bone and joint pain. The emotion it is associated with is fear, and the patient may come to us with his fears. Since there are kidneys and bladder at the root of the tree, it may also present with organ complaints such as impotence, dysuria, and enuresis.

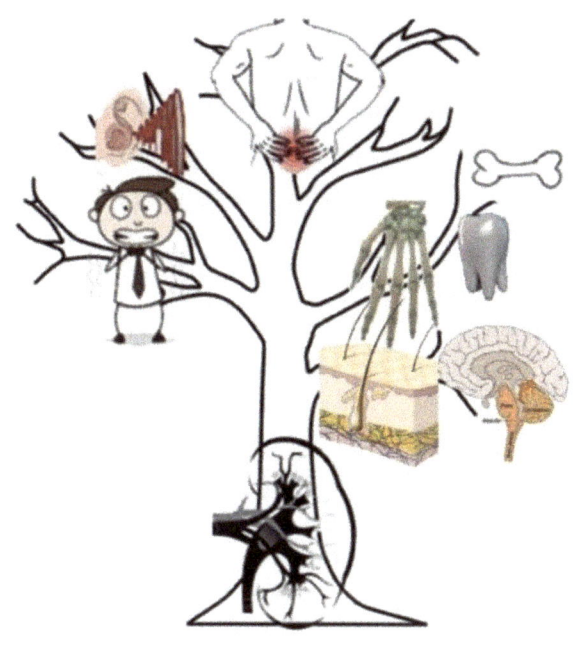

Figure 2: Kidney tree

The science of acupuncture requires a holistic perspective. When there is an energy imbalance in the water element, the patient may go to a physical therapist with musculoskeletal pains; to an otolaryngologist with complaints such as buzzing in the ear, hearing loss; to a psychiatrist with phobias, to a dentist with toothache; to a urologist with complaints of enuresis or impotence. If a physician in any of these specialties is also an acupuncturist, he/she can relieve the patient's complaints related to his/her own branch, as well as relieve complaints related to other branches.

A good acupuncturist focuses on treating the root of the tree by accurately assessing the symptoms and signs in the patient. For example, in a patient with low back pain, local injections to the painful area and relieving the patient's symptoms are considered as branch treatment. Of course, it is important to relieve the patient's back pain at that moment, but while doing this, the root cause of this pain should be found and root treatment should be done with points that balance the energy. He knows that in a patient who has only branch treatment without root treatment, the symptom that disappears may reappear after a short period of time, or even if the same symptom does not appear, it may manifest itself differently in different branches of the tree. For example, a patient who receives only dental intervention without root treatment may experience relief from toothache, but then complaints of hearing loss or tinnitus in the ear, which is located in the other branch of the kidney tree, may occur.

Acupuncture is the art of eliminating the blockage in the meridians and the energy imbalance in the organs by using certain acupuncture points. The five shu points are the most important points that we can do root therapy on the patient, that balance the energy, and these points and the logic with which they are used in the treatment will be explained in the following passages. Of course, in addition to the five shu points, there are many other point groups that balance energy such as luo yuan points, xi-cleft points, back shu points, front mu points, but in our book we will try to explain how to do this work through the five shu points.

DEFINITION OF THE FIVE ELEMENT THEORY

The Chinese equivalent of the five elements is Wu: five, Xing: dictionary meaning movement, process, behavior, but over time it began to be used to mean element. The dictionary meaning indicates that the elements are not passive and inert, but dynamic and dynamic. For this reason, it is also referred to as the five phase theory in some sources. The five elements theory states that the five elements, namely "Wood, Fire, Earth, Metal and Water" are the basic materials that make up our material world and that these elements are in a relationship with each other to maintain balance.

The yin-yang theory and the five element theory represent a historical leap in medicine from the view that disease is caused by evil spirits to the naturalistic view that disease is caused by lifestyle. The five element theory attempts to explain the physiological functions and pathological disorders of organs and tissues by observing the laws of the universe and interpreting how these same laws are manifested in the human body. This approach is in line with our religious and cultural heritage. Sheikh Galip expresses the meaning I want to say very well in the following couplet:

"Look kindly upon your essence that you are the essence of the world

You are Adam, the apple of the eye of existence"

In short, it is meant to be said that Adam is the essence of the universe. The laws that take place in the universe are manifested in the same way in Adam because of the unity of the Creator. For example, he looks at the effects of wind in the universe and tries to interpret how the same effects are manifested in the human body. The wind appears paroxysmally and then suddenly disappears. Just like this, in diseases such as asthma, epilepsy, migraine with paroxysmal attacks, he suspects the presence of internal wind. Based on the observation that the wind vibrates the trees in the universe, he suspects the presence of wind in diseases and symptoms such as convulsions, tics, tiremor with excessive mobility in the body. He likens the fact that the wind knocks down trees when it turns into a hurricane to the symptoms of block symptoms such as hemiplegia and facial paralysis, which are characterized by excessive immobility in the body. Another characteristic of the wind is that it is mobile. Therefore, in the presence of wandering lesions such as urticaria or wandering pain, he suspects internal wind.

The topic can be extended further by citing examples of similar approaches. Moisture tends to collapse due to its weight, while heated air rises. As can be understood from this analogy, dampness is usually the etiological cause of diseases in the lower half of the body such as back and knee pain, while heat dominates in diseases in the upper half of the body such as migraine.

Although this approach may seem primitive at first glance to those of us who have studied modern medicine, there is nothing more natural than a medical system that dates back thousands of years to approach diseases in this way. My advice to students who are just starting their acupuncture education is to learn and practice this system in the same way as it came to us. The Western Medicine approach and the TCM approach are very different from each other. An approach such as "anti-inflammatory points are used in the presence of inflammation, immunomodulatory points are used in immunodeficiency" without removing the Western Medicine glasses while evaluating diseases will not take you beyond being a point acupuncturist.

HISTORY OF THE FIVE ELEMENT THEORY

The first source on the five elements dates back to the Zhou dynasty (ca. 1000-771 BC). The theory of the five elements was applied not only in medicine but also in astrology, natural sciences, calendar, music and even politics. From a historical perspective, it is an important pillar of medical theory and one of the main diagnostic and treatment protocols. In modern clinical practice, the five elements theory is used in different ways depending on the practitioner and the style of acupuncture they are practicing.

Ancient philosophers who interpreted Nature in the light of Yin-Yang and the Five Elements and drew political conclusions from it were highly respected and perhaps somewhat feared by Chinese rulers. For example, each ruler is associated with a particular element, and ceremonies must match the color and season of that particular element. These philosophers claimed that they could predict successive rulers by referring to the various cycles of the five elements. During the rise of Huang Di [Yellow Emperor], large worms and large ants appeared. It follows from this that the earth element is in the rising sign, their color should be yellow and their work should be placed under the earth sign. During the ascension of Yu the Great, plants and trees that did not fade in autumn and winter appeared, from this it was concluded that the tree element was in the ascendant, our color should be green and our works should be placed under the tree sign. In the early first century, critical approaches to the five elements began to emerge. Wang Chong (AD 27-97) criticized the five-element theory for its rigid interpretation of all natural phenomena. During the Han Dynasty (206 BC-AD 220), the effectiveness of the five element theory in Chinese Medicine began to decline. For example, in the famous Chinese Medicine classic "Discussion of Cold-borne Diseases" written by Zhang Zhong Jing during the Han Dynasty, the five element theory is not mentioned at all. During the Song Dynasty (960-1279), the Five Element theory regained popularity. Starting from the Ming Dynasty (1368-1644), the five-element theory lost popularity again. During this period, Chinese Medicine was dominated by the study of disease pattern identification according to the four levels and triple heaters, which were used for the diagnosis and treatment of infectious diseases caused by external heat.

As we can see, the entire content of Traditional Chinese Medicine did not emerge in a narrow part of history and was transmitted to us in that way. In certain periods, the five elements theory was popular, in certain periods it fell out of favor, and then it was back on the agenda. During the periods when it fell out of favor, there were developments in different areas of Traditional Chinese Medicine.

INTRODUCTION TO FIVE ELEMENT THEORY

Let's start the topic with a quote from the Yellow Emperor. "An ordinary physician who does not know the basics of medicine and does not have knowledge of the five elements and Qi, without any knowledge of how the changes in the universe are applied in medicine, wastes his time, remains addicted to prescriptions, and harms people."

I think the Yellow Emperor's sentence "He is addicted to prescriptions" refers to both prescriptions for medicines and prescriptions for points. A physician who does not know the yin yang balance and the five element theory will have to ask someone else who he thinks knows better than him about the points he should use in every disease he encounters, and he will not be able to avoid becoming a point acupuncturist. Don't get me wrong, I say this as a person who knows that the door to knowledge is asking questions. There will and must be many cases in which we, as physicians, will consult each other and exchange ideas about diseases. When we look at the sources, you will see many cases where the authors contradict each other in some diseases. In fact, as you will understand better when we get into the subject, you will witness that the authors contradict each other even in diagnosing which pool is faulty, which is the first of the 3 steps in the approach to diseases. Our aim is to convey this job to you as we understand it, to teach you and to learn at the same time while teaching. The easiest way to learn this job is to practice and experience acupuncture on yourself, just as you do it on your spouse, friend and patients. It is obvious that there are different levels of knowledge that can be achieved by describing or showing baklava or making it taste to someone who has no idea about baklava and has never seen or tasted baklava before. Of course, the person who knows baklava best is the one who tastes it.

Just like this, when you apply acupuncture on yourself and observe its effects, you will learn this science much better. For example, if you have a headache, when you use certain acupuncture points, if there is an increase in the intensity of the pain, what caused this increase, if the pool I chose was hot, did I heat it even more or if it was cold, did I cool it even more, it will be much easier for you to comment on yourself and the result will be much more efficient and permanent. In an application that you have done wrong and caused complaints to increase, when you stop the application, you will see that the increased complaint returns to its previous state in a short time, and you usually do not cause permanent harm to the patient. I say "usually" because keep in mind that sometimes if you misjudge the pool, there is also the possibility of unwanted permanent consequences. For example, in a hypertension case where the pool is hot, when you heat the pool even more, the patient's hypertension may increase even more and you may leave a sequelae such as stroke. You should not ignore such a possibility, even if it is low, and you should know that everything that has an effect can also have side effects.

THE FIVE ELEMENTS AND THE CONCEPTS RELATED TO THEM

According to the five element theory, each element has an associated organ, sensory organ, tissue, emotion, season, environmental factor, taste, color, sound, spirit, music, grain, direction and numbers (Table 1). Since these have important aspects regarding diagnosis and treatment, they will be examined one by one.

Table 1	WOOD	FIRE	EARTH	METAL	WATER
ORGANS	LIVER GALL BLDDER	HEART-SMALL INTESTINE PERICARDIUM - SANJIAO	STOMACH-SPLEEN	LUNG-LARGE INTESTINE	KIDNEY BLADDER
SENSORY ORGAN	EYE	TONGUE	MOUTH	NOSE	EAR
TISSUE	TENDON, NAIL	VESSEL	MUSCLES	SKIN, BODY HAIR	BONE, TEETH, HAIR, MEDULLA SPINALIS, BRAIN, SMALL JOINTS
FEELING	ANGER	JOY	OBSESSION	SADNESS	FEAR

[23]

SEASONS	SPRING	SUMMER	LAST 18 DAYS OF EVERY SEASON	AUTUMN	WINTER
ENVIRONMENTAL FACTOR	WIND	HEAT	DAMPNESS	DRYNESS	COLD
TASTE	SOUR	BITTER	SWEET	ACRID, TART	SALTY
COLORS	GREEN	RED	YELLOW	WHITE	BLUE-BLACK
SOUNDS	SHOUT	LAUGHTER	SINGS IN STYLE	TEARFUL	GROAN
SOUL	HUN	SHEN	YI	PO	ZHI
SMELL	STINKING MEAT OR URINE	BURNED	FRAGRANT ODOR	STINKING MEAT, GARBA	STINKING MEAT, URINE

				GE TRUCK	
MUSIC AND SHEET NOTES	JUE (Mİ)	ZHİ (SOL)	GONG (DO)	SHANG (RE)	YU (LA)
GRAIN	WHEAT	WHİTE MİLLET	MİLLET	RICE	BEAN
DIRECTION	EAST	SOUTH	CENTRE	WEST	NORTH
NUMBERS	3,8	2,7	5,10	4,9	1,6

ORGANS

According to the five element theory, organs are represented by certain elements. The liver and gallbladder are represented by the wood element, the stomach and spleen by the earth element, the lung and large intestine by the metal element, and the kidney and bladder by the water element. While each element represents two organs, the fire element represents four organs. These are heart, small intestine, pericardium and sanjiao (Table 1). Every organ has a sister organ. The liver is a sister organ to the gallbladder, the heart to the small intestine, the sanjiao to the pericardium, the stomach to the spleen, the lung to the large intestine, and the kidney to the bladder. Since energy transfer occurs through deep connections between sister organs, the energy change in one of them passes to the sister organ in a short time, and when balance is reached, the energy transfer stops. For this reason, the energy appearances of sister organs are the same. For example, in a patient with lung Yin deficiency, in addition to the lung-related dry cough symptom, constipation, which is usually a large intestine related symptom, is also observed.

The functions of some organs differ from Western Medicine. For example, since the spleen is a sister organ to the stomach, it is responsible for digestion and absorption, takes part in the transport and transformation of fluids, keeps the organs in place, and keeps the blood in the veins. For this reason, fluid retention in the body, organ prolapse and spontaneous bleeding may be observed in spleen insufficiency. The pericardium protects the heart against external pathogenic factors. It is not considered an independent organ by some and you may see articles titled 5 zang -6 fu organ. The reason for this is that the author of the book does not see the pericardium as an independent organ. Sanjiao is a virtual organ that represents the cavities in the body. The space between the heart and lungs is called the upper jiao, the space around the stomach and the surrounding area is called the middle jiao, and the space around the bladder and uterus is called the lower jiao. All cavities in the body, such as the joint cavity, eye cavity, ear cavity, belong to sanjiao. Wang Ju Yi, a recent writer, even includes the interstitial area in sanjiao.

SENSE ORGANS

The eye is the sensory organ associated with the tree element. The first target that should come to our mind in all kinds of eye-related diseases such as visual disturbances, eye itching, eye dryness, and eye discharge will be the liver and gallbladder. The tongue is the sensory organ related to the fire element. The first target pool that should come to our mind in all kinds of language-related diseases such as lisping, aphasia, stuttering, aphtha on the tongue will be the heart, small intestine, pericardium and sanjiao. The mouth is the sensory organ associated with the earth element. When we say mouth, we should think of lips, buccal mucosa and gingiva. Our target pool for mouth-related diseases such as dry mouth, aphtha in the buccal mucosa and gingiva, dryness and cracks in the lips will be the spleen and stomach pool. The nose is the sensory organ associated with the metal element. For this reason, it is important to use the nose and not the mouth when breathing. In people who constantly breathe through their mouth, lung qi deficiency occurs over time. In all kinds of nose-related diseases such as odor disorders, nasal dryness, runny nose, nose bleeding, our target pool should primarily be the lungs and large intestine. Finally, the sensory organ associated with the water element is the ear. In case of any ear-related disorder such as hearing loss, ringing in the ear, earache, the primary pool that we should think of will be the kidney and bladder pool.

FEELINGS

According to the five element theory, each organ has an emotion associated with it. Just as pathologies in the organs can cause the emotions they are associated with, emotions can also directly cause disease in the organs. You can think of these as internal pathogenic factors. Excessive or insufficient emotions may cause disease in the associated organ. A balanced emotion does not harm the organ, on the contrary, it is beneficial for that organ. For example, it is normal for people to feel pain when they lose someone. Anger helps people assert their rights, and fear protects them from danger. The goal is the appropriate emotional response. When emotions last for a long time, become intense, repressed, or unacknowledged, they can cause an imbalance in a person's energy. Anger is an emotion associated with the liver. The liver pool is thought to be hot in people who are extremely angry. People with liver yin deficiency shine quickly, just like a small amount of water in an electric kettle boils quickly. Joy is the emotion associated with the heart. Insufficiency or excess of joy creates problems for the organ. An example of this is when a person has a heart attack after receiving overly joyful news. Obsession and excessive thinking are related to the earth element. In those with obsessive-compulsive disorder, the target pool is the soil pool. Sadness is the emotion associated with the metal element. If the patient states that his current complaint arose after losing a relative, you should keep in mind that the target pool may be the metal pool. Fear is the emotion associated with the water element. Fear, especially at a young age, can slow growth, cause hair loss, shorten lifespan, and even cause diseases in the bone marrow (such as leukemia).

According to TCM, while the brain is tissue related to the water element, its functions belong to the heart. Since Shen, translated as mind, is located in the heart and the task of evaluating and integrating all emotions belongs to the heart, all emotions actually affect the heart as well as the organ they are related to (Figure 3).

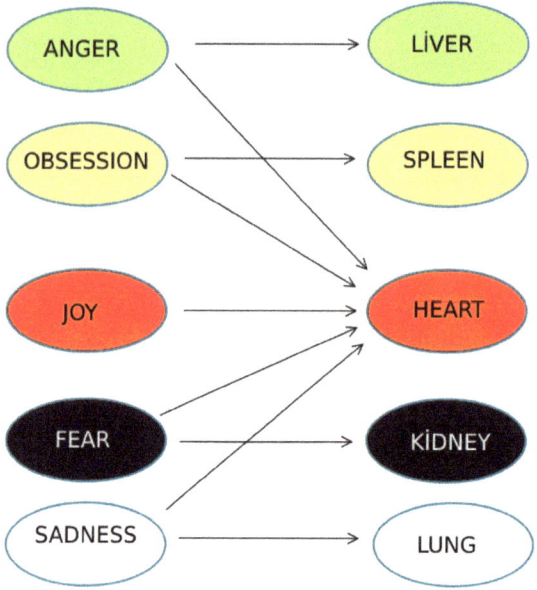

Figure 3: Organs and emotions

SEASONS AND ENVIRONMENTAL FACTORS

Each element has a season to which it is associated and an environmental factor to which it is more sensitive. The season associated with the wood element is spring, when trees begin to bloom. The environmental factor to which it is most sensitive is wind. The season associated with the fire element is summer, and the environmental factor to which it is most sensitive is heat. The season associated with the metal element is autumn, and the environmental factor to which it is most sensitive is dryness. Alveoli need moisture for healthy oxygen exchange in the lungs. The season associated with the water element is winter, and the environmental factor to which it is most sensitive is cold. During winter or cold weather, you often see an increase in patients' complaints of lower back pain and widespread joint pain. Although the season associated with the earth element is mentioned as the end of summer in some sources, it does not have a season. The last 18 days of each season belong to the earth element. Since the earth element is an important part of our postnatal energy, it is important to have a healthy stomach and spleen energy balance during the change of seasons in order to have a smooth adaptation to the new season. The environmental factor it is most sensitive to is humidity. You will often see that diseases related to the earth element are common in workers who live in humid geography, whose homes are in the basement, or who have to work in water or mud for long periods of time.

This does not mean that each element gets sick only in the season it is associated with or is affected by the environmental factor it is associated with. Of course, there is the possibility that each element will be affected by a season with which it is not related or by an environmental factor with which it is not related.

FLAVORS

According to the five element theory, each element has a flavor associated with it. The wood element is associated with sour taste. The fire element is associated with bitter taste. The earth element is associated with sweet taste. In some sources, the taste associated with the metal element is described as acrid and sour, and in some sources it is described as a sharp or spicy taste. The water element is associated with salty taste. While each taste benefits the organ it is associated with, excessive intake can cause harm. For example, while a balanced intake of sweet foods is beneficial to the earth element, excessive intake is harmful. Unfortunately, the disadvantage here is that the boundaries of "balance" and "extremism" cannot be defined. We can say the same for all elements and the flavors they are associated with.

Huangdi Neijing notes that after a meal, sour-flavored foods go first to the liver, bitter foods go first to the heart, sweet foods go first to the spleen, spicy foods go first to the lungs, and salty foods go first to the kidneys. This information has an important clinical aspect. Knowing that spicy foods go to the lungs first, consuming spicy foods, especially in winter and cold weather, can help the lungs remove pathogenic factors such as wind and cold from the body. Based on the knowledge that salty tastes first go to the kidneys, the recommendation to take some herbal formulas necessary for the treatment of the kidneys with some salt water becomes understandable.

COLORS

According to the five element theory, each element has a color associated with it. The wood element is associated with the color green. It is also mentioned as blue in some sources. The color turquoise, which is a mixture of shades of green and blue-green, is also considered within the scope of the tree element. The fire element is associated with red, the earth element with yellow, the metal element with white and grey, and the water element with black. Colors help us in both diagnosis and treatment. We are all aware of the blackish color tone seen in dialysis patients. Likewise, knowing the color tone associated with each element will help us in diagnosis. Knowing the colors of the elements also helps us in treatment. For example, in case of an energy imbalance in the liver, suggestions such as consuming green plants or painting the patient's room green will contribute positively to the recovery of the disease. You can think of a similar example for other elements as well.

SOUNDS

When we hear a person's voice, we can understand his situation. There have been many people in history who have been able to do this. There have been physicians who were able to understand the nature of the patient's illness when he spoke, even while behind a wall. Because tones of voice and disease are related to each other. A shouting, angry tone of voice indicates the wood element. The element of fire comes to mind in a cheerful person who laughs out loud at everything that happens between his conversations. The singing voice tone suggests the earth element. This tone of voice is similar to the tone of voice that occurs when singing a lullaby to a baby or soothing a sick person. A tearful tone of voice indicates the metal element, and a moaning tone indicates the water element.

SOULS

According to the five element theory, each element has a spirit associated with it. Let's examine the clinically important aspects of these together.

PO (CORPORAL SOUL)

It is the spirit of the lungs. It enters the body at birth and dies when the body dies. It is the aspect of the soul that is related to the physical body. Good breathing causes Po to take root in the body. It activates the Essence in all physiological processes. Essence is motionless without Po. Po is the mediator between the other vital substances of the body and the Essence. The Essence enters and exits all parts of the body through the Corporeal Spirit. It plays a role in all physiological activities of the body. This means that whenever we are going to tonify the Essence, it is better to also strengthen the Corporeal Spirit. This information explains why the confluent point of the ren meridian, which nourishes the Essence best, is on the Lung meridian, and why the complementary point is on the kidney meridian (LU-7 Lieque and KI-6 Zhaohai).

Because of the relationship between the Bodily Soul and the lungs and its conjugate organ, the large intestine, the anus is also called the "gate of the Po". Therefore, the BL-42 Pohu ("Po's Window") point is indicated for cases where both urine and feces cannot be retained due to fear. Considering the connection between the Bodily Soul and death, the ellipsis related to the lungs (DU12, UB13, UB42) is used in those with suicidal thoughts (Figure 4)

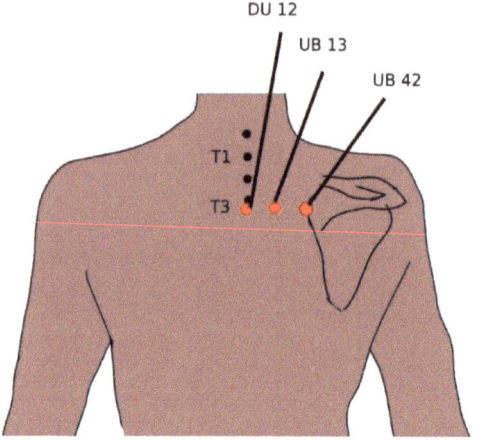

Figure 4: Points aligned with the lung back shu point

The Corporeal Soul gives us the capacity to feel, hear and see. When the Corporeal Spirit is developed, the ears and eyes become sharp. Decreased hearing and vision in older people are caused not only by the decline of renal essence, but also by the weakening of the bodily soul.

SHEN

It is the soul belonging to the heart, but it is like the overseer and leader of other souls. In the sources, Qi, Essence and Shen are called the three treasures. Essence and shen are states of Qi in different concentrations. Essence is the most concentrated form of Qi, while Shen is the most dilute form (Figure 5) Shen is the treasure we do not share with animals. Animals have Essence and Qi but not Shen. Shen is what gives people human consciousness. Thought, consciousness, self-identity recognition, perception and feeling of emotions, sleep, intelligence, and idea generation can be counted among the functions of Shen.

THREE TREASURES

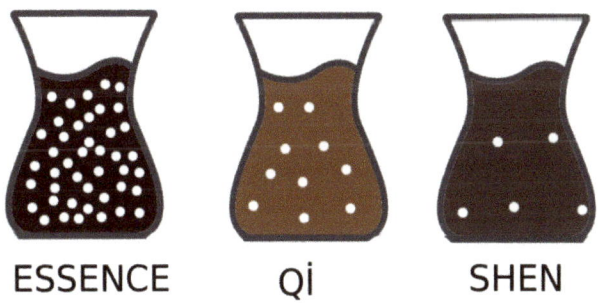

Figure 5:Three Treasures

If Shen is healthy, falling asleep is problem-free and short-term memory is strong. The disease is reflected in the clinic in ways such as difficulty falling asleep, not knowing why we came to the room, not being able to remember the name of someone we just met, and forgetting where we put our belongings. Shen's condition can be understood by the brightness of the person's eyes and whether he makes eye contact with people.

HUN (ETHERIC SOUL)

It is the spirit of the liver. It is said that Hun enters the body at birth and leaves the body when the person dies and continues on its way (Figure 6).

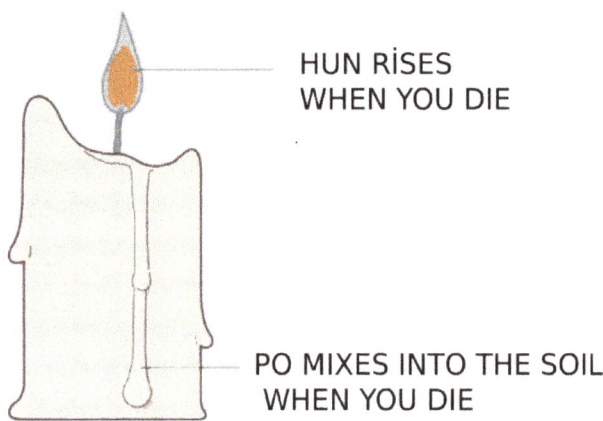

(Figure 6: Hun and Po's situation with death)

Hun is associated with people's ability to realize their life plans and have spiritual vision or insight. When it flows into the eyes during the day, vision; When it flows into the eyes at night, the dream comes true (Figure 7). Interestingly, most dreams occur during rapid eye movement (REM) periods.

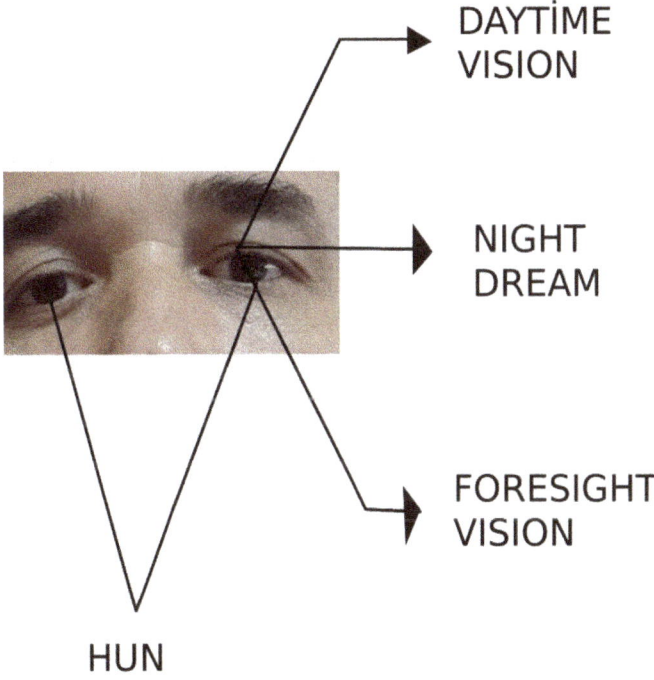

Figure 7: Hun and eye relationship

Dreams speak to us in a symbolic language because they originate from Hun, not Shen. In the presence of a liver disease that prevents Hun from being retained in the liver, sleepwalking or a trance state may occur. If a person constantly experiences vague and confused dreams, it may be due to an imbalance affecting the Hun in the Liver.

The Etheric Soul is responsible for our capacity to relate, interact, and empathize with other people. Therefore, it can be said that autism is a pathology of the Etheric Spirit. This information belongs to Giovanni Macciocia. Radha Thambirajah interprets autism as a disease of the heart. In the previous passages, I said, "You will witness that even the authors contradict each other in diagnosing which pool is faulty." This issue is one of them.

If there is inadequate flow to and from Hun Shen, as in Liver-Qi stagnation, it can cause depression or autism; if it oscillates excessively (as in Liver-Yang rising or Liver-fire), the person may become agitated, angry, or very emotional, or may exhibit some degree of mania and cause hyperactivity (Figure 8). The Etheric Spirit is related to courage, and its deficiency is related to cowardice. When the Etheric Spirit is not strong, one becomes timid.

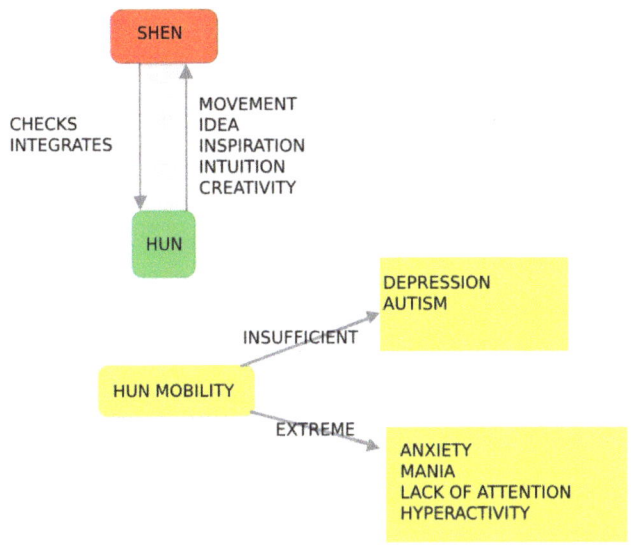

(Figure 8: Etheric soul and Hun relationship)

Since Shen is immature in children, he cannot suppress Hun sufficiently. They live in the etheric spirit world, a wild world of imagination and fantasy where inanimate objects come to life. Behaviors that are normal in children may be considered mental illness in adults. After about age 7, Shen matures and begins to control Hun. In a coma, Shen is completely incapacitated and therefore unable to function, yet the person is not dead. This means that there are other mental aspects as well. These are the Etheric Spirit and the Corporeal Spirit. In fact, for death to occur, not only Shen must die, but also the Etheric Soul must leave the body and the Corporeal Soul must return to the earth.

ZHI

Zhi is the spirit associated with the kidneys. It is usually translated as will or impulse. It gives the drive to reproduce and thus ensure the survival of the species and the family. Zhi gives us the driving force or drive that keeps people motivated to achieve things in life. People with weak kidneys also have a weak vitality. It is Zhi's duty to store and memorize data. It is Zhi's job to store data that dates back a long time ago.

Yİ (İNTELLECT)

It is the spirit associated with the spleen. There is a very close relationship between the Yi of the Spleen and the Shen of the Heart. It can be said that Yi is nothing but a sub-aspect of Shen. Therefore, Yi is the part of Shen that allows us to memorize data, study, concentrate and focus. There is a relationship of mutual dependence between Yi and Shen. Yi needs Shen's direction and coordinating activity, and Shen needs Yi for memorization, concentration, and focus. It is responsible for thinking, studying, memorizing, focusing, concentrating and generating ideas. If the spleen is weak, the Mind will become dull, thinking will be slow, memory will be poor and studying, concentration and focus will be poor.

In the area of memory, there is significant overlap between the intellect (Yi of the Spleen), mind (Shen of the Heart), and Willpower (Zhi of the Kidneys). The main distinguishing factor is that the Spleen is responsible for memorizing data, especially during one's work or study. It is not uncommon for a person to have a brilliant memory in the field of study or research (a function of the Spleen), but to be quite forgetful in daily life (a function of the Heart and Kidneys).

SMELL

According to the five elements, each element has a scent associated with it. Since people's perception of smell is different, the description of these smells varies in the source books, but they are the smell of wood and water elements, rotten meat and urine. The smell of the fire element is the smell of burning. The smell of the earth element is referred to as fragrant odor. This is probably the translation that expresses what is meant in the worst way possible. This smell is generally unpleasant. It is described as the smell of fermented millet. It is also described as the nauseous smell of rotten fruit, newborn vomit, a bakery or a bad perfume that permeates the nostrils and the room for a long time. You may also see different definitions for the metal element, such as the smell of stinky meat or a garbage truck.

If a patient has a strong odor, this is evidence of heat dominance in that organ. If there is a strong odor in the stool, there is heat in the intestines, if there is a strong odor in the urine, there is heat in the bladder, if there is a strong odor in the armpit, there is heat in the heart or liver, and if there is a strong odor in the mouth, there is heat in the stomach. Bad breath may be due to lung and kidney heat as well as stomach heat. You may have difficulty establishing the connection between kidney heat and bad breath. If you remember that teeth are a tissue belonging to the water element and know that tooth decay is an important cause of bad breath, the uncertainty in your mind will disappear.

MUSIC AND SHEET NOTES

TCM believes that music moves and vibrates blood vessels, allowing the essence and spirit to circulate. The Chinese characters for music and herbal medicine are very similar (Figure 9).

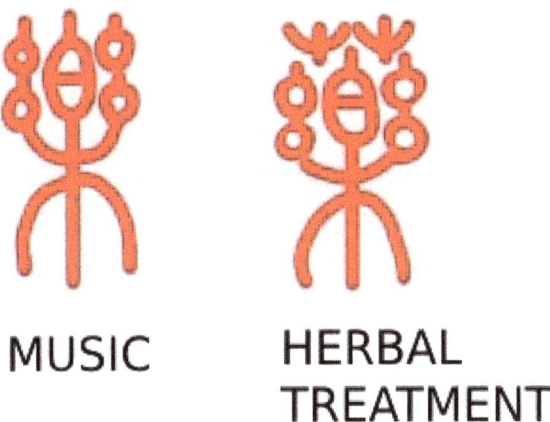

Figure 9: Chinese character of music and herbal medicine

Generally translated as notes in source books, jue (Mi) is related to the wood element, zhi (Sol) is related to the fire element, gong (Do) is related to the earth element, shang (Re) is related to the metal element, and yu (La) is related to the water element.). As far as I understand, it refers to either a tone of voice or a musical style rather than a note. These musical styles, in which the elements are related, were used in the treatment of organ diseases. Since this area requires a little more research, let's leave it at that.

GRAİNS

According to the five element theory, each element has a grain that is associated with it. Wheat is the grain associated with the tree element, white millet with the fire element, millet with the earth element, rice with the metal element, and beans with the water element. The bean resembles a kidney and perhaps for this reason it is a grain belonging to the water element. Legumes and legume products have a particularly strong effect on the kidneys and the bones and brain with which the kidneys are associated. A dietary supplement derived from legumes that has recently become popular is lecithin. In China, lecithin is used to regulate blood fats, improve cerebrovascular functions, improve memory and reduce hair loss. Among grains, rice is the grain of the lungs, and the lungs are associated with skin and body hair. Therefore, rice has a cosmetic effect. It can be thought that one of the reasons why the hair and skin of people living in the south of China are more beautiful than those living in the north is that rice is used as the main grain material in the south of China and wheat in the north.

DIRECTIONS AND NUMBERS

According to the five element theory, each element has a direction it is related to. The east is associated with the wood element, the west with the metal element, the south with the fire element, and the north with the water element. The earth element does not have a specific direction, it is located in the center (Figure: 10)

Although I scanned many sources about the relationship of elements with directions, I could not find much data addressing their importance in the field of Medicine. Let's say a few words about this in order to open the door to the mind and encourage those who are interested in the subject to research. A science called Fengshui emerged on the basis of the relationship of elements with directions. As far as I can see, this science has developed mostly in home decoration today. When you type "Home decoration according to Fengshui", you will see many articles about this on the websites. Considering that the north direction is associated with the water element and that the water element is associated with cold, one of the seasonal factors, it seems reasonable to place the head of the bed in the north direction. Because the most Yang side of the body is the head and the most Yin side is the feet, the Yang side of the body will be balanced with the Yin direction, and the Yin side of the body will be balanced with the Yang direction.

According to the five elements, each element has a number associated with it. The number 1 is associated with the water element and the north, 2 with the fire element and the south, 3 with the wood element and the east, 4 with the metal element and the west. The number 5 is associated with the earth element and is located in the centre. To create a second number sequence, 5 is added to these numbers. So when 5 is added to the number 1, it becomes 6. In this case, the numbers 1 and 6 are related to the water element, 2 and 7 to the fire element, 3 and 8 to the wood element, 4 and 9 to the metal element, and 5 and 10 to the earth element (Figure 10). The numbers associated with the elements were generally used in astrology.

Although there is information in the sources that the ancients used numbers to adjust the formulas of herbal medicines, the number of medicines and the dosage of each plant, unfortunately, I could not find detailed information about this science.

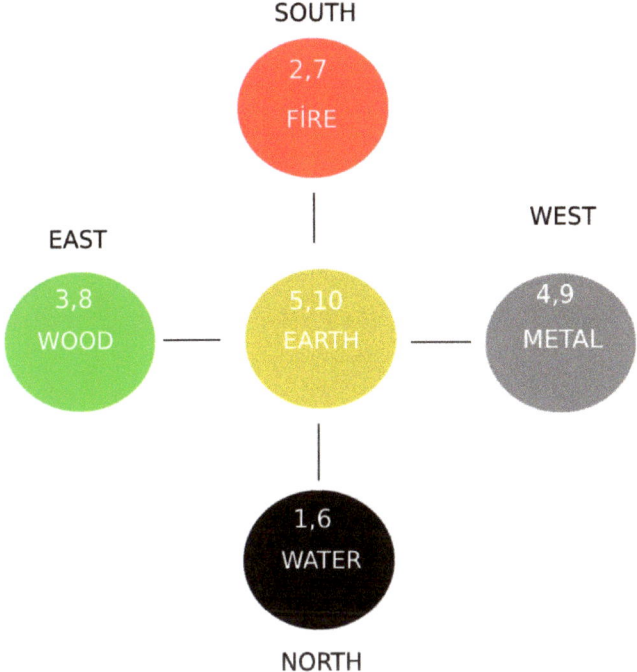

Figure 10: Elements and associated directions and numbers

MUTUAL RELATIONSHIPS OF THE FIVE ELEMENTS

There are mutual energy transitions between organs. While some of these energy transitions have physiological effects, some have pathological effects. In order to understand the physiopathology of diseases, we will examine this mutual interaction between organs under four headings.

1. Mother and son interaction (Sheng cycle)
2. Controlling interaction (Ke cycle)
3. Excessive suppressive interaction
4. Degrading interaction

1. MOTHER-SON INTERACTION (SHENG CYCLE)

We said that the five element theory states that the same laws that occur in the universe are also in force in humans. The tree burns and fire appears. So the tree feeds the fire. The fire burns to ashes or the fire heats the ground. Therefore, fire nourishes the earth. The soil stores and grows minerals in it. Therefore, soil nourishes metal. Metal nourishes water with minerals. Water also nourishes the tree. This interaction between elements is equally valid between organs, and this interaction is called by different names such as mother-son interaction, nurturing interaction or reproductive cycle (Figure 11).

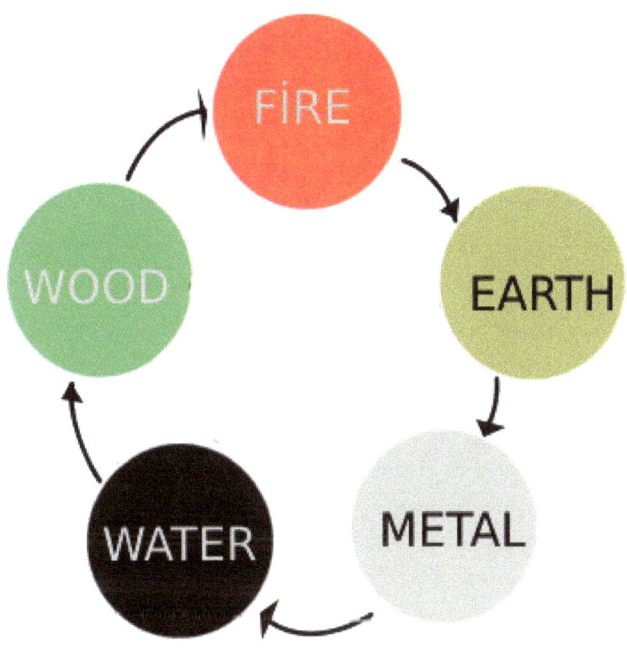

Figure 11: Mother and son interaction

(Sheng cycle)

In this interaction, the wood element is the mother of the fire element and the son of the water element. The fire element is the son of the tree element and the mother of the earth element. The earth element is the son of the fire element and the mother of the metal element. The metal element is the son of the earth element and the mother of the water element. The water element is the son of the metal element and the mother of the wood element. The parent element nourishes the son element. From the Yin organ of the parent element to the Yin organ of the son element; Energy flows from the Yang organ of the parent element to the Yang organ of the child element. Just as the disease in the mother can affect the son, the disease in the son can also affect the mother.

Let us give a patient example for a better understanding of the subject. I decided to use points on the meridians of the organs belonging to the earth and metal elements in the treatment of a patient who had been suffering from frontal headache and purulent postnasal drainage intermittently for years. How I decided on these meridians is a subject I have not yet explained, but the reason will be better understood after the following passages. Then I noticed a skin lesion extending from the sole of the patient's foot to the medial aspect of the leg (Figure 12).

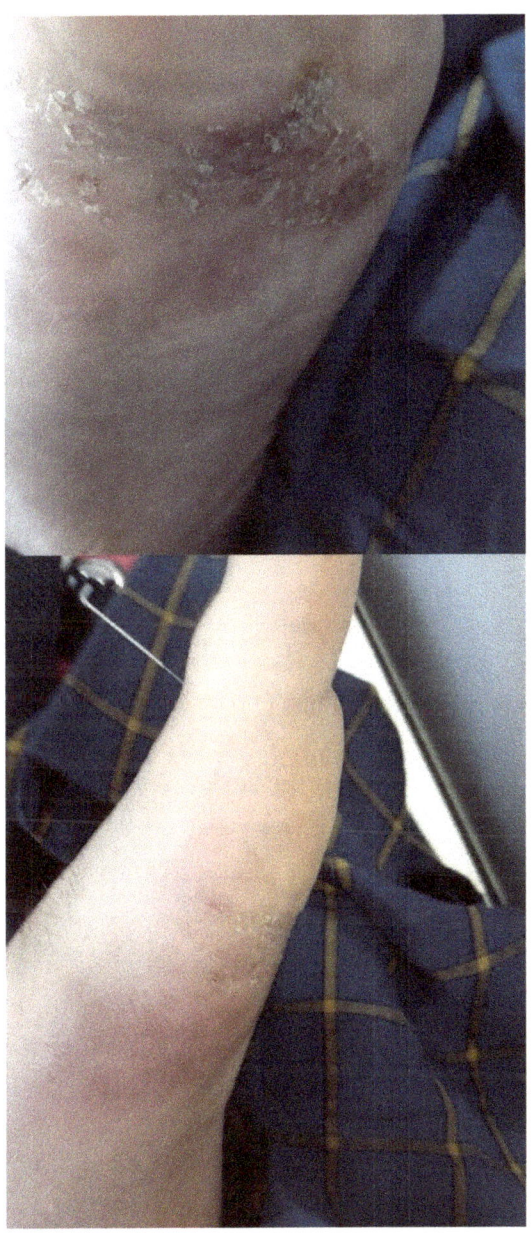

Figure 12: Skin lesion following the kidney meridian course

When I enquired, he reported that this lesion had been present for many years. As a result of the investigations into the cause of the lesion, the treatment given did not yield any positive results. The lesion on the patient's foot was along the course of the kidney meridian. While the lesion was prominent on the foot, its course on the leg was indistinct. In this patient, if you treat only the organs belonging to the earth and metal elements and do not treat the water element, which is the son of the metal element, the success rate of your treatment will decrease.

2. CONTROLLER INTERACTION (KE CYCLE)

We said, "For each element, the previous element becomes its mother and the next element becomes its son." In this case, each element has a grandmother two rows before and a grandson two rows after. For example, while the mother of the tree element is the metal element, its grandson is the earth element. It is based on the principle that the grandmother suppresses her grandchild. Fire melts metal, earth attracts water, metal cuts wood, water extinguishes fire, wood pierces the earth (Figure 13). Another name for this interaction between organs is suppressive interaction. Both mother-son interaction and controlling interaction are physiological interactions. This mutual interaction between the elements is essential for maintaining the natural balance in the body. In the mother and son cycle, energy transfer occurs from Yin organ to Yin organ, and from Yang organ to Yang organ, while in the controlling cycle, energy transfer occurs from Yin organ to Yang organ, and from Yang organ to Yin organ. For example, if the Yin of the water element is insufficient, it cannot suppress the Yang of the heart and empty heat rises in the heart. This is the mechanism of menopausal hot flashes.

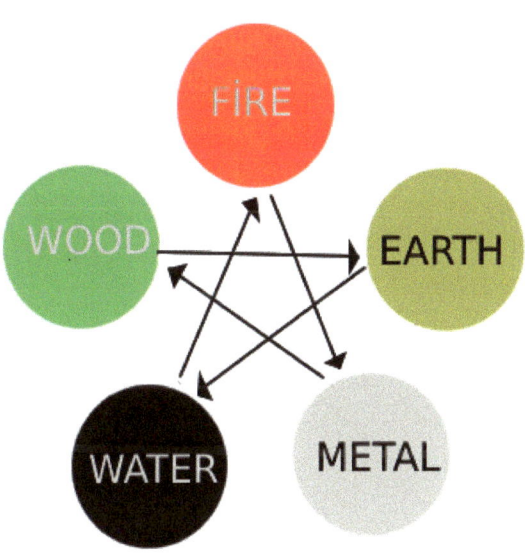

Figure 13: Controlling interaction

3. EXCESSIVE SUPPRESSIVE INTERACTION

In an overly suppressive interaction, the energy flow is from the grandmother to the grandson, just like in the controlling interaction. The grandmother's suppression of her grandchild was a physiological effect. If this suppression is excessive, it causes disease (Figure 14). For example, in a person who is nervous during a meal may experience indigestion if the wood element overpresses the earth element, which is its grandson. For this reason, Chinese Medicine does not recommend eating while angry. The reason for nausea and vomiting in migraine patients before or during the attack is that the increase in Yang in the wood element over-suppresses the earth element and disrupts the downward gastric Qi flow. In the presence of an excess of dampness in the earth element, it may over-suppress its grandson, the water element, and cause the patient to have damp-type low back pain in the morning or ear pain due to otitis.

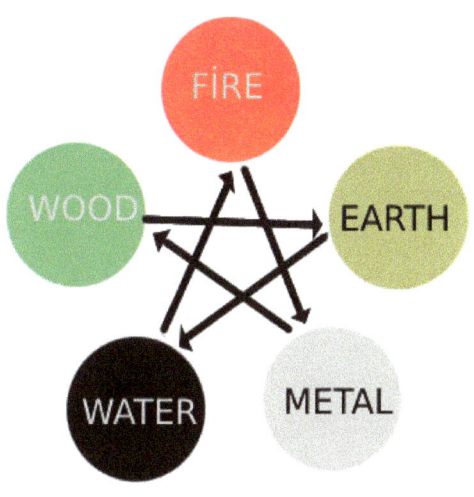

Figure 14: Over-suppressive interaction

4. İNSULTİNG INTERACTION

In a insulting interaction, the energy transfer is from the grandchild to the grandmother. In physiological interaction, the grandmother should suppress the grandchild, but here, on the contrary, the grandchild suppresses the grandmother, which is called the grandchild's humiliation of the grandmother (Figure 15). This is also a pathological situation. For example, gallbladder fever can suppress the descent of lung Qi and cause asthma or urticaria. If the bladder cannot adequately excrete fluids, the spleen may be affected. Small intestinal fire may spread downward and cause renal Yin deficiency.

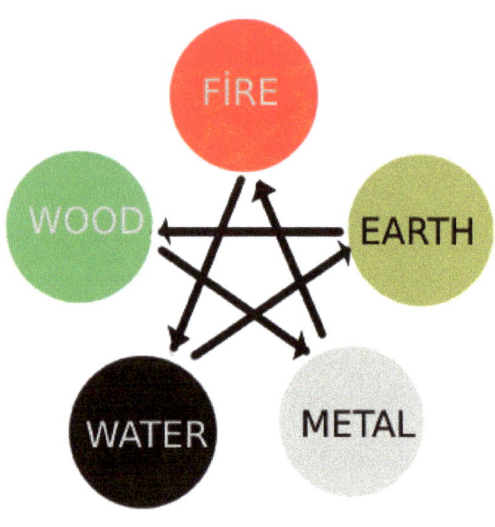

Figure 15: İnsulting interaction

A question may come to mind here: Why does the state of excess in the element not over-oppress the grandchild, but humiliate the grandmother? For example, in some cases of hepatitis in the liver, itching occurs on the skin. We give this as an example of a case where the grandchild (wood) insults the grandmother (metal). In this case, it can be asked why the tree element does not over-oppress its grandchild but humiliates its grandmother. Energy has a tendency to flow from high places to low places. In the hepatitis example we gave, if there is no weakness in the lungs, but the stomach energy is weak, the energy may flow towards the stomach instead of the lungs and cause nausea and vomiting.

It is important to consider these four interactions in order to understand the physiological and pathological energy transitions between organs and thus the physiopathology of diseases. Sometimes it may be difficult to decide whether the grandmother over-repressed the grandchild or the grandchild humiliated the grandmother. Although this situation is not clinically very important, the decision is made according to which element the complaint has arisen first. For example, if a patient who develops gastroenteritis develops conjunctivitis shortly afterwards, you can say that the grandmother suppressed the grandchild excessively. If conjunctivitis developed first and then gastroenteritis developed, you can say that the granddaughter humiliated the grandmother. In any case, the metal and wood element organs will be sedated. There may be an advantage in knowing this. If the grandmother overpressed the grandchild, it is usually sufficient to sedate only the grandmother. If the grandchild has humiliated the grandmother, it will be sufficient to sedate only the grandchild. If both organs are sedated, this will not be a problem. Anyway, if such cases are usually treated correctly, they will recover quickly with one or two days of treatment, and sedation will not be necessary for a long time.

In addition to these four interactions, the arrangement of the elements, which we mentioned when describing their orientation, should also be taken into account in the treatment. Giovanni calls this placement of the elements cosmological placement (Figure 16).

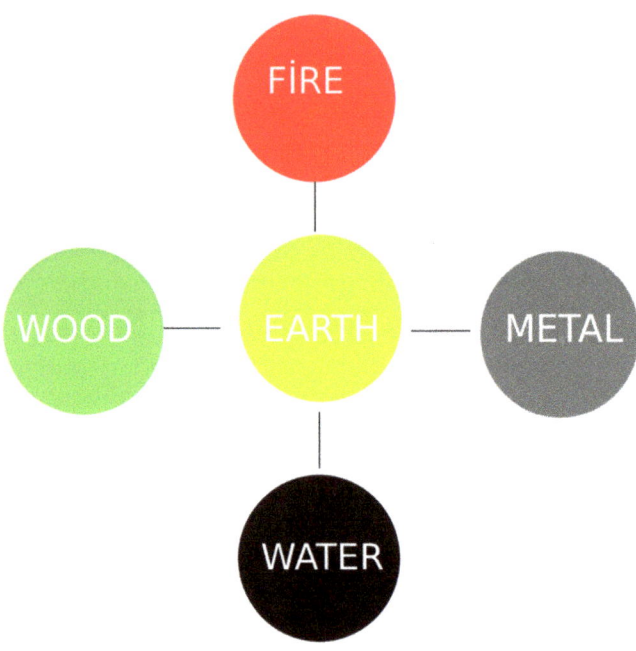

Figure 16:Cosmological arrangement of the elements

Since the earth element is located in the center in this type of settlement, it is the mother of all elements. In other words, we understand that in case of any organ failure, points on the stomach and spleen meridians can be added to the treatment on the relevant meridian of that organ

CRITICAL APPROACHES TO THE FIVE ELEMENTS THEORY

Both Giovanni Macciocia and other authors have criticised the five element theory, and in this section of the book we will discuss two of these criticisms. The criticisms concerning the five shu points will be addressed later in the book.

FIRST CRITICISM:

"The eyes are related to the liver. While it is true and important in practice that the liver moisturises and nourishes the eyes, it is not the only organ that affects the eyes, and not all eye problems are related to the liver. For example, kidney Yin also moisturises the eyes and many chronic eye problems are related to the kidneys. The heart also reaches the eyes through the luo channel. Some acute eye problems, for example acute conjunctivitis, are usually not related to any organ but are caused only by external Wind-Heat. Many other channels are associated with the eyes, for example the lungs, small intestine, gall bladder and triple heater".

ANSWER TO THE FIRST CRITICISM:

The five element theory looks at the sense organs to which the elements are related as part of a system. Since it sees the eye as part of the liver and gall bladder system, it considers a case of conjunctivitis due to hot wind as a reflection of an energy imbalance in this system. The same applies to the other sense organs. For example, the five-element theory does not say, "Cases of otitis are usually not related to any organ, but are caused only by the external wind-cold". Since it sees the ear as a part of the kidney and bladder system, it considers a case of otitis due to cold wind as a reflection of the energy imbalance in this system. I wonder if Giovanni would have made the same comment if we had looked at the subject not with the five elements theory, but with the four-level classification of infectious diseases related to external heat, which was popular during the Ming Dynasty (1368-1644). In other words, would he have said "Acute conjunctivitis is usually not related to the four-level classification, but is only caused by external Wind-Heat"? I think he would probably attribute this case to the Qi phase, which is one of the phases of the four levels, and to the gallbladder heat, which we can call the sub-phase of the Qi phase. Since this sentence I have formed is outside the content of the book, it may not be understood for the reader who is unfamiliar with the subject. Those who are curious about the details can investigate the four-level classification of hot pathogens. I do not see Giovanni's statement "The liver is not the only organ that affects the eyes" as a criticism of the five element theory. Because the five element theory does not say such a thing anyway. He says that the eye is a sensory organ associated with the tree element, but the organs can affect each other through interactions such as mother-son interaction, grandmother-grandchild interaction.

SECOND CRITICISM:

"The five element theory associates the Liver with the eyes, the Kidney with the ears, and the Spleen with the muscles. This may be useful in clinical practice, but as such, one-to-one correlation is no longer valid. For example, if a woman suffers from blurred vision and, in addition, has poor memory, infrequent menstruation, drowsiness and dizziness, we can say that the liver blood does not nourish the eyes: this case therefore confirms the relationship between the liver and the eye in the theory of the five elements. But if the same woman suffers from dry eye and glaucoma, as well as lower back pain, vertigo, tinnitus and night sweats, this tells us that the kidney-Yin is not moisturizing the eyes. Therefore, the second case falls outside the five-element model."

ANSWER TO THE SECOND CRITICISM:

In the second criticism, it is said in summary: If the complaints accompanying the eye problem are liver-related symptoms, it is easy to attribute the eye problem to the liver, but if the accompanying symptoms are related to the kidney element, this does not comply with the five element theory. The five element theory interprets that if eye-related symptoms are accompanied by symptoms related to kidney Yin deficiency, water cannot nourish the wood. In this case, it nourishes both the Yin of the kidney and the Yin of the liver.

In a vast sea, the situation of a captain with a clear route and a captain with an uncertain route is not the same. The five element theory gives us a route. For example, if you have a complaint about your eyes, it says you should head to the wood element pool. But be careful, if the accompanying symptoms also indicate a different organ, it says change your route to that organ after the liver (Figure 17).

FİVE ELEMENT THEORY

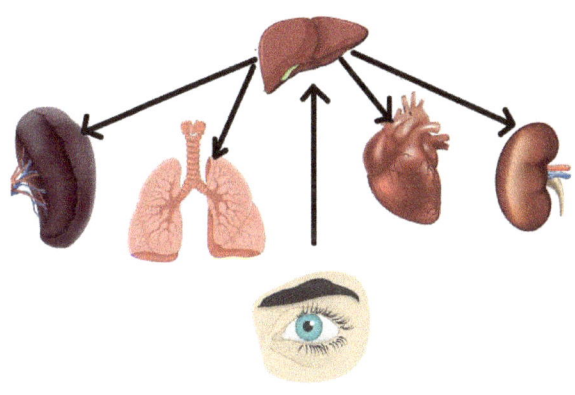

Figure 17: Example of a captain with a clear route

It is obvious that the five element theory provides great convenience in the acupuncture approach. I am not saying that this system should not be criticized because it provides convenience. We can all find it reasonable that a system that dates back thousands of years and whose effectiveness has been experienced by its practitioners may have been mixed with some superstitious information until it reached the present day.

Right and wrong are evaluated, wrong information is discarded and we continue with the correct information.

The five element theory approach helps us a lot in finding the broken pool. In the following passages of the book, it will be explained which parameters we will use to find the broken pool. Tongue and pulse examination, which are among these parameters, is a difficult process that takes time to learn, especially for those new to acupuncture. The situation of a student who is trying to find the broken pool, who does not know the five element theory and who is just at the beginning of this path, is similar to the situation of the captain whose route is unclear, as we have just given an example (Figure 18).

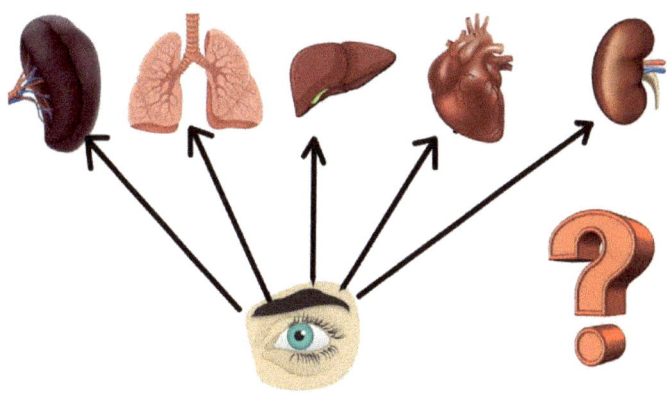

Figure 18: Example of a captain whose route is unknown

ENERGY VİEWS OF SISTER ORGANS AND THEIR RELATED MERIDIANS

We have previously said that the energy appearances of sister organs are the same, that there is energy transfer between them through deep connections, that the energy change in one of them passes to the sister organ in a short time, and that the energy transfer stops when balance is reached. We can think of sister organs as a combined container or as two pools with a transition between them. We can compare the meridians, which carry energy to sister organs, to a fountain of cold and hot water (Figure 19).

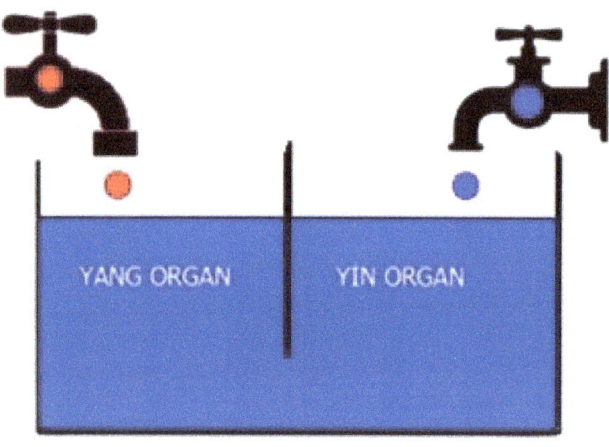

Figure 19: Sister organ and meridian metaphor

Although the energy appearances of sister organs are the same, the energy appearances of sister meridians are not the same. Let's take the metal pool as an example. While the energy appearances of the large intestine and lung, the sister organs of the metal pool, are the same, the energy appearances of the large intestine meridian and the lung meridian are not the same. Since one is a cold water fountain and the other is a hot water fountain, more Yang energy flows through the large intestine meridian and more Yin energy flows through the lung meridian. The energy appearances of all Yang meridians are not the same. In other words, the temperature of all hot water fountains is not the same (Figure 20). Just like some underground thermal water resources are extremely hot, some are at medium temperature, and some are at low temperature.

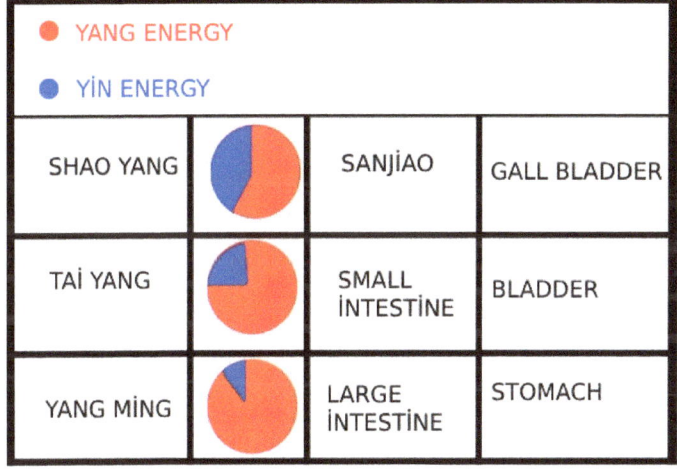

Figure 20: Yin-Yang ratio in Yang meridians

We say the same thing for the Yin meridians. The energy appearances of all Yin meridians are not the same. Some are extremely cold, some are moderately cold, and some are slightly cold (Figure 21).

SHAO YİN	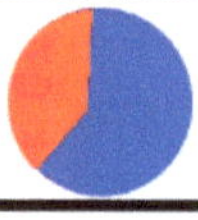	HEART	KİDNEY
TAİ YİN	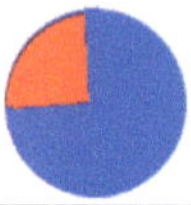	LUNG	SPLEEN
JUE YİN	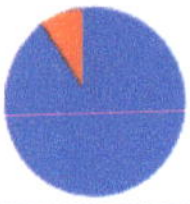	PERİCARDİUM	LİVER

Figure 21: Yin-Yang ratio in Yin meridians

I took these tables from Thambirajah and also included them in my book "Systematic Acupuncture". According to these tables, the meridians with the highest Yang energy are the Yang Ming meridians, that is, the large intestine and stomach meridians. In other words, the fountains that flow the highest degree of hot water are the large intestine and stomach fountains. The meridians where Yin energy is most intense are the Jue Yin meridians, that is, the liver and pericardium meridians. In other words, ice cold water flows through the liver and pericardium meridians. This discourse contradicts the quotes of western writers. Some scholars, such as Giovanni and Claudio Focks, say that Yang energy is most concentrated in the Tai Yang meridians, and Yin energy is most concentrated in the Tai Yin meridians. They say that the dictionary meaning of the word "Tai" is

"Great", so "Tai Yang" means "Great Yang" and "Tai Yin" means "Great Yin".

I think it is essential to clarify this issue in order to understand the effect of some acupuncture points and to understand some acupuncture issues. My personal opinion is that what Thambirajah said on this subject is correct, that is, the meridians with the highest Yang energy are the Yang Ming meridians, and the meridians with the highest Yin energy are the Jue Yin meridians. I will talk about two pieces of evidence that lead me to think so.

According to TCM, the disease potential of wind entering the body from the front or from the back is not the same. The wind entering the body from behind has been compared to an enemy attacking from behind and is seen as having a higher potential to cause disease. While Yang Ming meridians are located on the front of the body, Tai Yang meridians are located on the back. The energy that protects the body against external pathogens is Yang energy. If there was a higher amount of Yang energy in the Tai Yang meridians, the wind entering the body from behind would not be so feared, and the analogy of an enemy attacking from behind would not be made.

My second evidence will actually support the first evidence. In the famous Chinese Medicine classic "Discussion of Cold-induced Diseases" written by

Zhang Zhong Jing during the Han Dynasty, diseases are classified into six stages, and the first stage is the Tai Yang stage. Since the first phase is the Tai Yang phase, we understand that the cold pathogen enters the body from the posterior. As we said in the second evidence, if there was a higher amount of Yang energy in the Tai Yang meridians, the cold pathogen could not enter the body from the back. In this case, it could not be said that the first phase of the six phases was the Tai Yang phase.

So, in this case, what could be the reason why the Yang meridians passing from the back are called "Great Yang" and the Yin meridians passing from the front are called "Great Yin"? The front of the body is Yin, the back is Yang. If Yin meridians pass through the front of the body, two Yins overlap. Therefore, it deserves the name "Great Yin". If the Yang meridians pass through the back of the body, the two Yangs overlap. Therefore, it deserves the name "Great Yang".

TERMINOLOGICAL INFORMATION

I will soon explain how I apply five element acupuncture in the clinic, in a very clear and understandable manner, through representations. Before getting into the subject, I would like to explain the terms Yin dominant and Yang dominant, which will be used occasionally in the book. When I use the Yin dominant term for a disease, you will understand that the pool is cold. There may be different reasons why this pool is cold. Either the cold water fountain is overflowing (excess case), which is also called full cold. Either the hot water fountain is flowing insufficiently (deficiency case), which is called empty cold. Or both the hot water fountain is flowing insufficiently and the cold water fountain is flowing excessively (deficiency and excess together). Of course, there may be other possibilities other than these three. For example, both fountains flow excessively together, but the cold water fountain is much more extreme. Or both may be flowing inadequately, but the hot water fountain is even more inadequate. When I say the pool is cold or the case is Yin dominant, it includes all of these possibilities.

Similarly, when I say the pool is hot or the case is Yang dominant, either the hot water fountain is flowing excessively (excess case), which is also called full hot. Either the cold water fountain is flowing insufficiently (deficiency case), which is called empty hot. Or both the cold water fountain is flowing insufficiently and the hot water fountain is flowing excessively (deficiency and excess together). Please also consider the different possibilities mentioned above. Even if we ignore the different possibilities, when you say the pool is hot, you understand that there are at least these three possibilities (Figure 22).

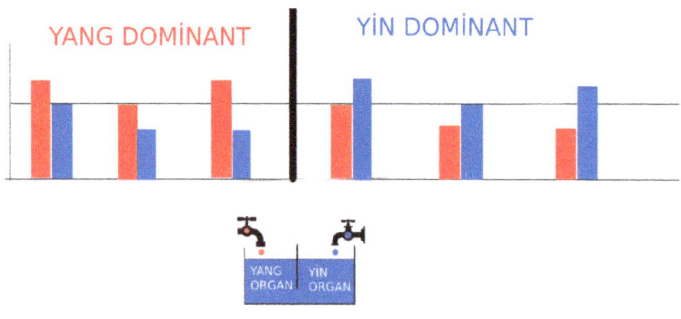

Figure 22: Energy images in hot and cold pool

THREE STEPS TO APPROACHING DISEASES

So far we have given general information about the five elements. In the next part of the book, I will try to explain how I apply five element acupuncture in the clinic. We physicians, trained in Modern Medicine, have a really hard time understanding TCM. We find it difficult to make sense of many abstract concepts. I've been thinking for a long time about how to simplify these abstract concepts. The best way to simplify this task and make it more logical is to use representations. I will try to convey to you, my readers, the five element acupuncture, which is difficult to understand and requires a long time, in the shortest possible way, by making it very easy to understand, through representations.

If you follow the three steps I will explain to every patient you encounter in the clinic, your success rate will be at its highest. In the first step, we will try to answer the question of which pool is faulty. In the second step, we will check the temperature of the faulty pool we found. In the third step, we will try to regulate the temperature of the pool using hot and cold water taps (Figure 23). Now let's consider these three steps one by one.

1. WHICH POOL IS DEFECTIVE?

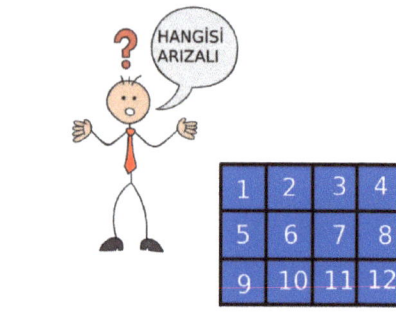

2. CHECK THE TEMPERATURE OF THE POOL

3. REGULATE THE TEMPERATURE OF THE POOL

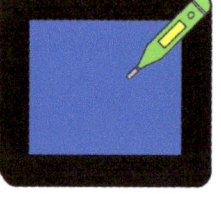

Figure 23: Three steps in approaching diseases

FIRST STEP

FIND THE FAULTY POOL

We will represent the organs in the body and the meridians of these organs with a pool. Since we have 12 organs and the meridians belonging to these organs, this means we have 12 pools in our target. First of all, we will find which of these pools is faulty (Figure 24). This first step is the most important step in the approach. A mistake here will invalidate the other steps.

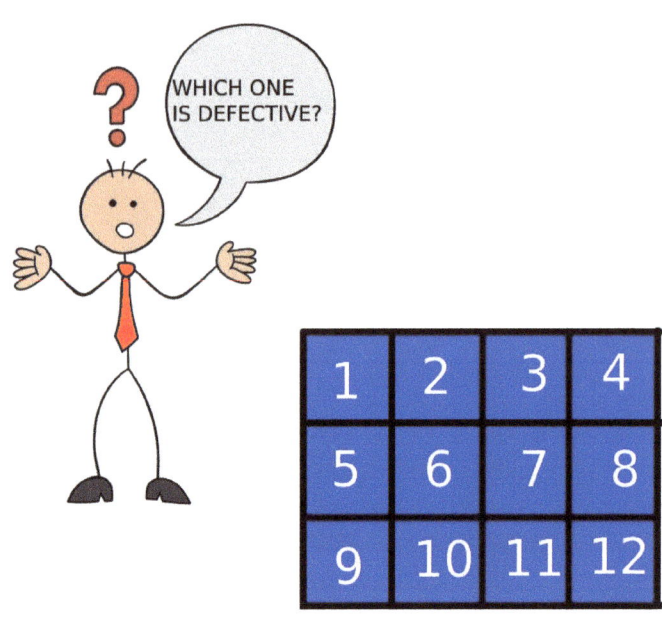

Figure 24: First step

In finding the faulty pool, the meridian course and complaint area, organ-specific symptoms, the sensory organs, emotions and tissues to which the organs are related according to the five element theory, tongue and pulse examination and author comments will help us (Figure 25).

- Meridian course
- Complaint area
- Organ specific symptoms
- Sensory organ with which the organs are related
- Tissue with which organs are related
- The feeling that the organs are related
- Tongue and pulse examination
- Western Medicine
- Authors' comment

Figure 25: Parameters to be used to find the faulty pool

MERIDIAN COURSE

Some of the patients we encounter in the clinic describe meridians very well. For example, he says he has a headache. When we ask where his headache is, he says it travels around the side of his head and extends to his toes. We understand that it describes the gallbladder meridian, and we call the faulty pool the gallbladder pool (Figure 26).

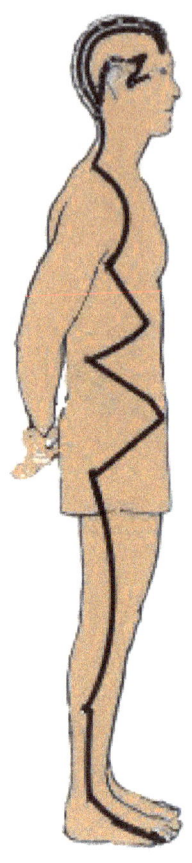

Figure 26: Gallbladder meridian course

Most patients do not describe the meridian in its entirety in this way, but describe a part of the meridian. For example, he says, "I have pain in my wrist, it extends to my thumb." We understand that it describes the lung meridian, we call the faulty pool is lung pool (Figure 27). If the complaint of extremity pain extends to the fingers, it is much easier to predict the course of the meridian. In order to understand the meridian course, the complaint does not always have to be pain; it may be numbness or a skin disease that follows the meridian course.

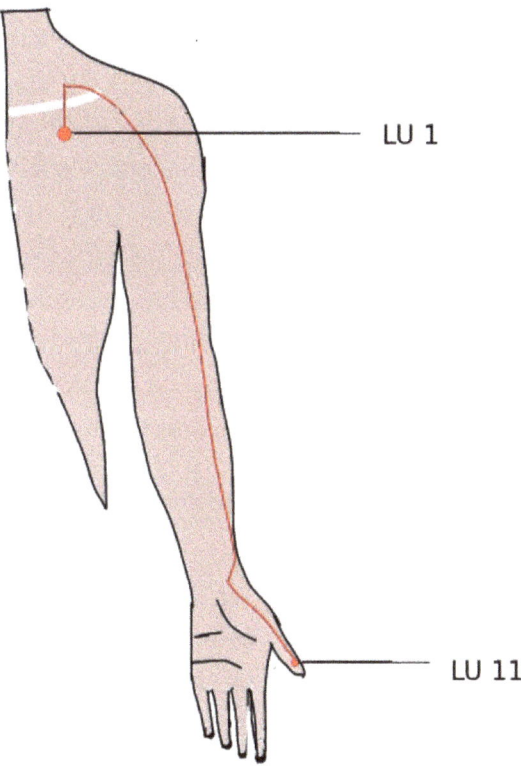

Figure 27: Lung meridian course

COMPLAINT AREA

The patient does not always describe a meridian course, as I said above, but an area. For example, the front of my head hurts, the back hurts. In such cases, first of all, the sensitive point is scanned by palpation and the meridian course is tried to be captured. If we are not sure, then we turn to certain meridians according to the area described. For example, if he says the front of my head hurts, it is necessary to turn to the meridians in the anterior of the extremities; if he says the back of my head hurts, it is necessary to turn to the meridians in the posterior extremities; if he says the side of my head hurts, it is necessary to turn to the meridians on the lateral side of the extremities (Figure 28). By the way, let me also point out that we cannot determine a direction for the top of the head. In such a case, treatment is performed through the wood pool. Headache here is just for example purposes. Our aim is to set a rule. Do not think that this approach is only applied to headaches; it is the same for all limbs. For example, in waist and back pain, the meridians on the posterior of the extremities are used for treatment, while in lateral thoracic pain, the meridians on the lateral side of the extremities are used. But there is a point to be considered here. If the disease is not a superficial disease related to the meridian course, but a disease related to the internal organs, there may be pain at the points where the organs are represented, which we call front mu and back shu points. Therefore, in the case of pain in the thoracic and abdominal region where the internal organs are located, decide on the defective pool together with the organ-specific symptoms that we will discuss in the next topic.

While explaining the mother-son interaction between the elements, I said that I planned to use points on the meridians of the earth and metal elements in the treatment of a patient with frontal headache. Now you understand better why I use the organs of earth and metal elements in frontal headache. Because meridians belonging to the metal and earth element are located in the anterior of the upper and lower extremities (Figure 28).

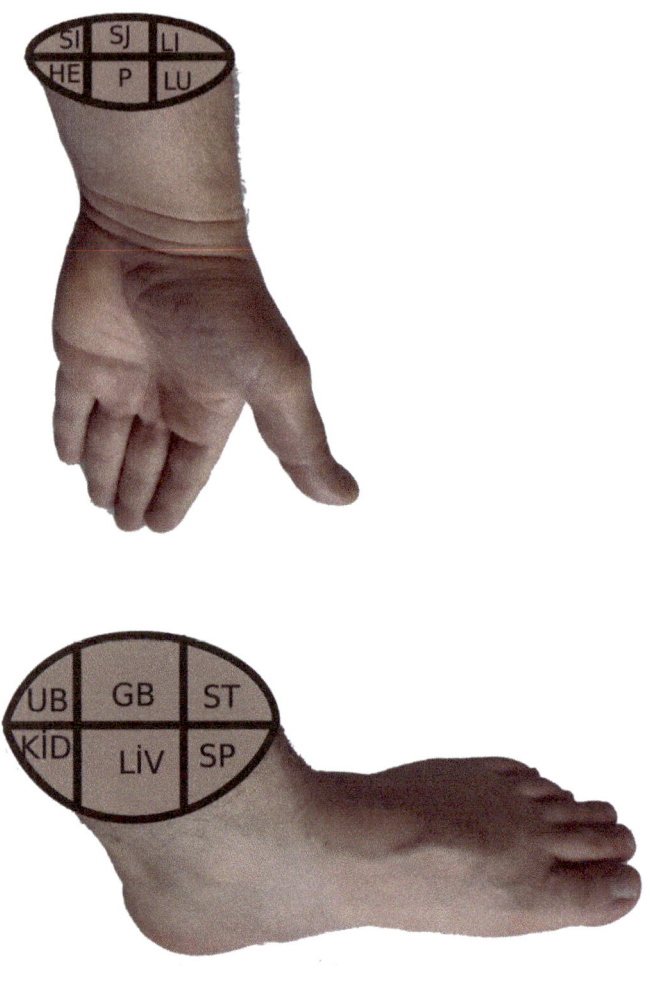

Figure 28: Transverse section of meridians located in the extremities

ORGAN SPECIFIC SYMPTOMS

The most important parameter in finding the faulty pool is organ-specific symptoms. While it is easy to find the faulty pool by looking at the meridian course and complaint area in superficial diseases such as musculoskeletal system diseases or skin diseases, in organ diseases, the most important parameter that will direct us to the faulty pool will be organ-specific symptoms. For example, complaints such as cough, phlegm, hoarseness, shortness of breath direct us to the lung pool. It directs symptoms such as palpitations, chest pain, and sleep disturbance to the heart pool. Complaints such as nausea, vomiting, and epigastric pain direct us to the stomach pool.

Symptoms such as constipation, diarrhea, and abdominal pain refer to the large intestine pool. Complaints such as urinary incontinence, burning in urine direct us to the bladder pool, etc.

Of course, it would not be right to head directly to a pool with a single symptom. It is necessary to evaluate all the symptoms of the patient together and make a decision accordingly. Symptoms may also indicate different pools, and in the clinic we often see multiple pools malfunctioning together.

Here, organ-specific symptoms should be understood as more than one symptom complex rather than a single symptom. For example, we said above that the symptom of insomnia among the symptoms points to the heart pool. Insomnia can actually be observed when the liver pool is malfunctioning. The fact that the symptom of insomnia was accompanied by palpitations and chest pain clarified our direction.

SENSORY ORGANS, TISSUE AND FEELINGS WITH WHICH THE ORGANS ARE RELATED

As a five element acupuncturist, of course the sensory organs, tissues and emotions with which the organs are related will guide us in finding the faulty pool. We have responded to Giovanni's criticisms on this subject in previous passages.

When treating a disease, we do not always have to go through the pool pointed by the sensory organ. For example, in cases of otitis in children, the Sanjiao meridian is mostly used in the treatment. However, the ear was the sensory organ related to the water element. According to TCM, since the kidney Essence is responsible for growth and development, treatment through the kidney meridian is not recommended due to the possibility of sedation of the kidney causing growth and development retardation in the child. The reason why we use the Sanjiao meridian is that the ear is located on the lateral side of the body. So, in this case, we are going to treatment through a different pool with the "Complaint area" instead of the "Sensory organ".

Similarly, we do not have to go to treatment through the pool pointed by the tissues. If you do not get a sufficient response from a treatment you perform through the pool indicated by the tissues, you can turn to a different pool. For example, a toothache is a very disturbing, severe pain and you need to relieve the patient very quickly. If you treated such a patient via the kidney and bladder meridian and could not relieve the patient's pain, you can change the pool via the "Complaint area". In other words, since the complaint area is in the anterior of the body, you can use the meridians in the anterior of the extremities.

Without trying treatment through the pool indicated by the tissues, you can also go directly to the pool indicated by the "complaint area". For example, in a patient with alopecia areata in the temporal region, since the hair is the tissue associated with the water element, you can also treat it through the kidney and bladder meridians. Since the temporal region is on the lateral side of the body, you can also use the meridians on the lateral side of the extremities (sanjiao, gallbladder and, if necessary, sister meridians). You can even combine both approaches.

Let's repeat the information we have given before, considering its importance. If you can follow the meridian course of the patient, keep the treatment secondary to the tissues to which the organs are related. For example, in a skin disease that follows a meridian course, first treat it on that meridian. In other words, do not say that the skin, points to the metal pool and go first through the lung and large intestine meridians. Likewise, in case of muscle pain, first consider the treatment based on the meridian course and the "Area of Complaint". In cases where you cannot receive treatment through the meridian course or the "Complaint Area", such as fibromyalgia, you can use the spleen and stomach meridians by saying that the muscles are the tissue associated with the earth element.

In addition to what I said, you can also use emotions, smells, tastes, sounds and colors to find the faulty pool. I do not see the need to say anything additional to what I have said before about these.

TONGUE EXAMINATION

One of the most important parameters in finding a faulty pool is the tongue examination. Of course, it is not possible to cover the tongue examination in full detail in this short book. I would like to share with you the points that I see as important in the clinic. However, at this stage of the book, we will not evaluate the findings in tongue. Don't forget!

We are only at step one and trying to figure out which pool is faulty. In the second step, we will measure the temperature of the pool and evaluate the tongue findings.

Certain parts of the tongue, direct us to certain pools. The tongue root points to the water pool, the central part points to the earth pool, the lateral part along its length points to the wood pool, the anterior 1/3 part points to the metal pool and the tip points to the fire pool (Figure 29). I specifically conveyed it by element names, because my current opinion is parallel to the view that the organs are represented in the same localization of the tongue, together with its sister organ.

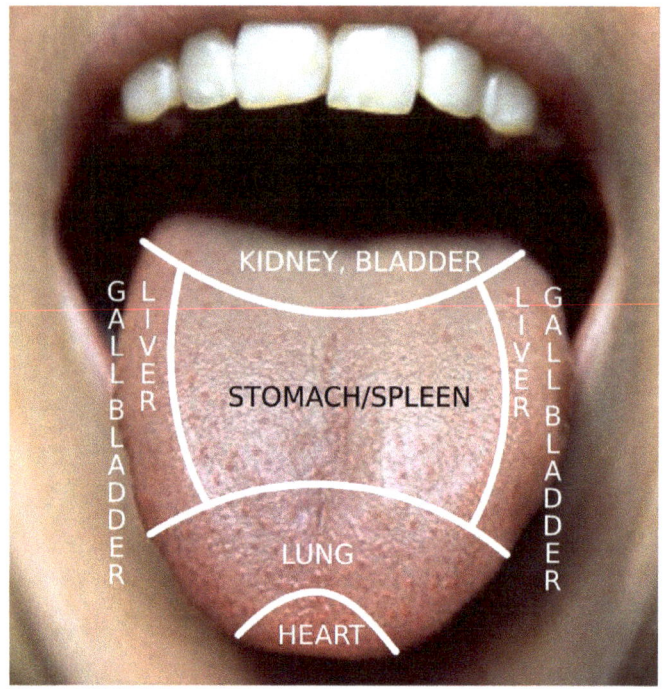

Figure 29: Representation areas of organs in tongue

There is also a different view that says that the intestines are also represented at the root of the tongue, as the front part of the tongue represents the upper Jiao, the middle part represents the middle Jiao, and the back part represents the lower Jiao. Therefore, do not be surprised if you see pictures in some sources showing that the intestines are also represented at the root of the tongue (Figure 30).

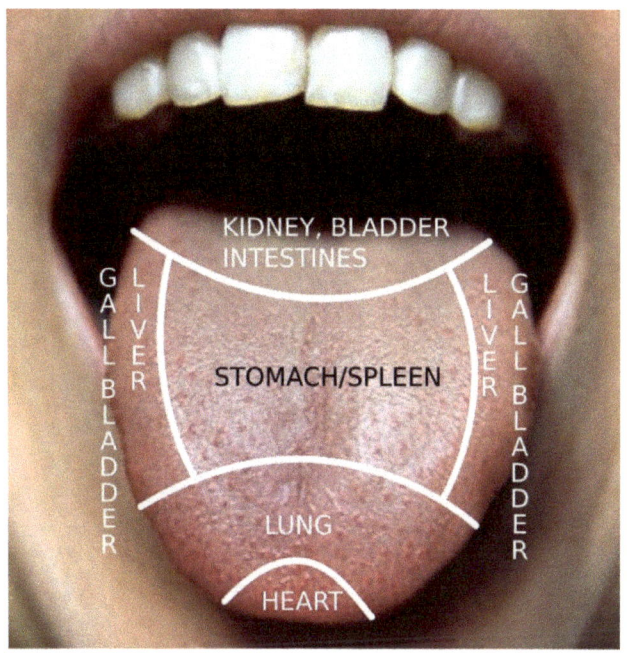

Figure 30: Representation areas of organs in tongue

We have said that sister organs are like communicating vessels, and that the energy change in one of them passes to the sister organ in a short time. Therefore, it seems more reasonable to represent sister organs in the same region of the tongue. Although Giovanni published a picture in his book in which the intestines are represented at the root of the tongue, I think he is of the opinion that the organs are represented in the same localization with his brother. Because when describing the tongue finding in the "full heat of the small intestine", he states that the tip of the tongue is hyperemic.

PULSE EXAMINATION

In the pulse examination, just like in the tongue examination, certain regions indicate a certain pool. The right hand points to the distal position metal pool, middle position to the earth pool, proximal position to the water pool (Figure 31).

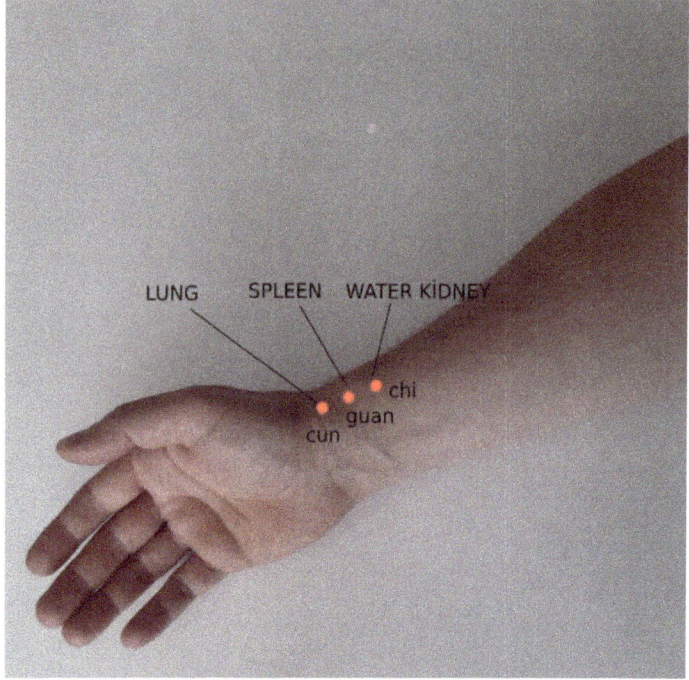

Figure 31: Right hand pulse positions

Left hand distal position points to the heart pool, middle position points to the wood pool, proximal position points to the water pool (Figure 32)

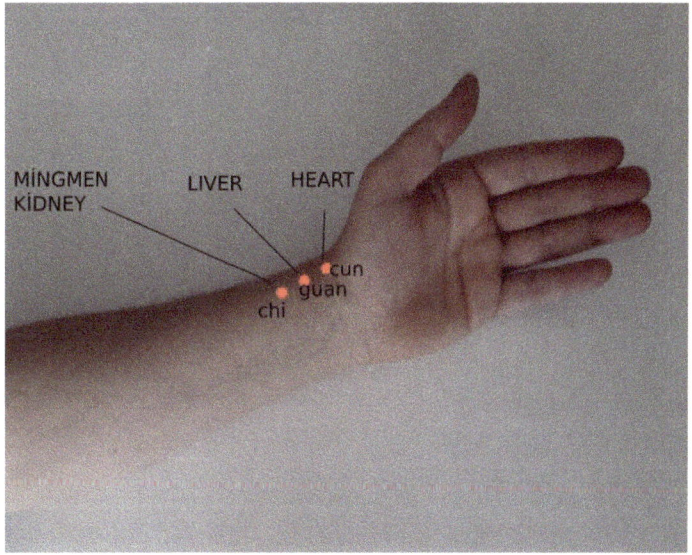

Figure 32: Left hand pulse positions

The evaluations I deem necessary regarding the pulse will be made in the second step. We are currently trying to find the faulty pool. Therefore, knowing the localizations where the organs on the wrist are represented will be sufficient for now. The position of the posterior pulse is a matter of dispute in the sources. Giovanni says that the right hand posterior represents the "Kidney Yang" and the left hand posterior represents the "Kidney Yin."

The view I adopt regarding the pulse is Thambirajah's view. Thambirajah quotes the left posterior pulse as "Mingmen kidney" and the right posterior pulse as "Water kidney". In fact, kidney Yin and Yang are checked from both wrists. In reproductive problems such as puberty, menstruation, libido, fertility and menopause, from the left side; She also recommends evaluating the kidney pulse from the right wrist in cases of non-reproductive kidney problems such as dryness, urination, edema, and bladder problems. In diseases related to the sensory organs, emotions and tissues that the water element is associated with, she recommends evaluating the right side posterior pulse.

WESTERN MEDICINE

We can also use Western Medicine to find the faulty pool. For example, in a patient with a diagnosis of hepatocellular carcinoma on tomographic examination, we can say that the faulty pool is the liver pool (Figure 33). Of course, it should be used in combination with the other parameters we use to find the faulty pool, keeping in mind that there may be interaction between the organs and that there may be problems in other pools along with the wood pool.

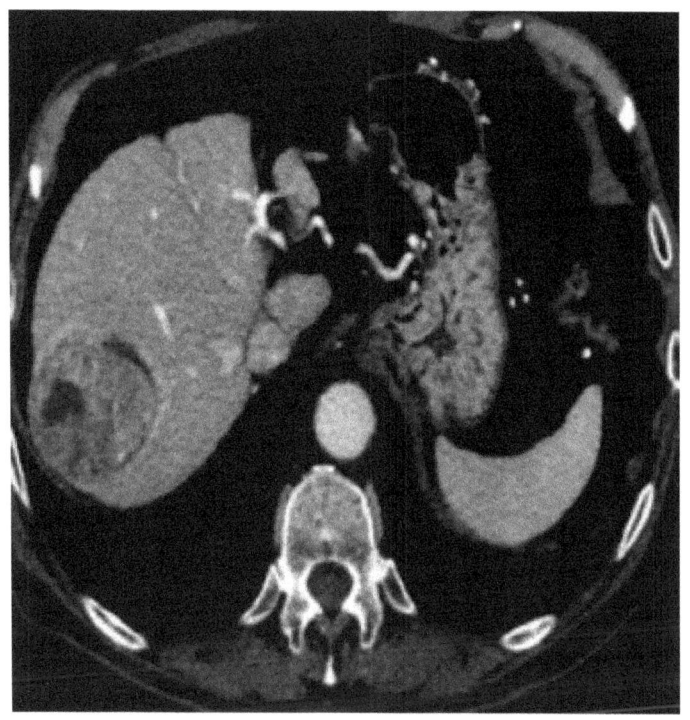

Figure 33: İmaging of hepatocellular carcinoma

AUTHORS' COMMENT

While there are so many parameters in finding the faulty pool, a question may come to mind: is there any need for an author's comment anymore? Sometimes, even though all parameters are used, it may be difficult to find the faulty pool. Since we, as Modern Medicine physicians, generally interpret the diseases diagnosed by Western Medicine according to TCM, we may disagree about which pool is the faulty one. For example, in diseases diagnosed by Western Medicine such as depression, anxiety, autism, restless legs syndrome, you will see that there is a lot of disagreement even among the authorities about which pool is the faulty one. For this reason, you should use all parameters together in diagnosis and make the final decision accordingly.

SECOND STEP

CHECK THE TEMPERATURE OF THE POOL

After using all the parameters and finding the faulty pool in the first step, it is time for the second step. In the second step, we will need to check the temperature of the pool we found (Figure 34). While checking the temperature of the pool, we will benefit from the patient's current symptoms, physical examination and the expert's comments.

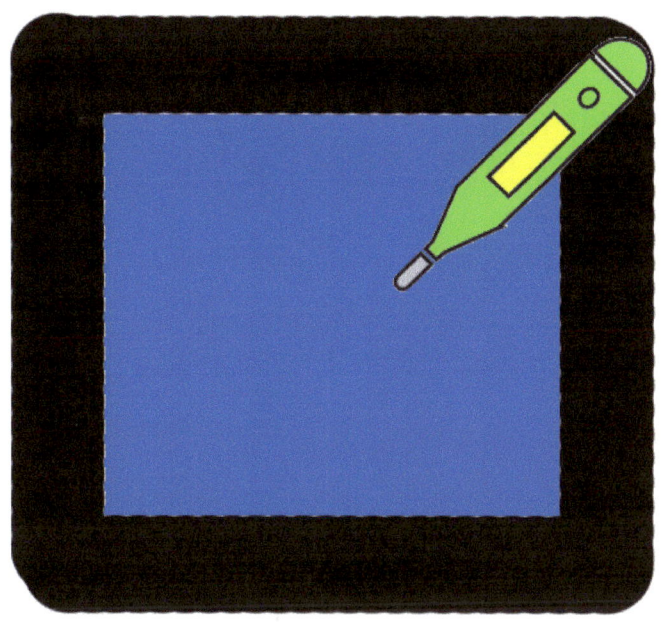

Figure 34: Second step, checking the temperature of the pool

SYMPTOMS

In the table below, you can see which symptoms indicate a hot pool and which symptoms indicate a cold pool (Table 2). The decision whether the pool is hot or cold can often be made based on symptoms alone. Of course, this decision is reinforced with the physical examination findings, which we will explain under the next heading.

Table 2: Hot and cold pool symptoms

HOT POOL	COLD POOL
DRY MOUTH AND DESIRE TO DRINK A LOT OF WATER	DESIRE TO DRINK VERY LITTLE WATER
PREFER COLD FOODS	PREFER HOT FOODS
DOES NOT LIKE NOISE AND LIGHT	NOISE AND LIGHT DO NOT CAUSE ANY DISTURBANCE
DRY EYE, DRY NOSE, DRY SKIN MAY OCCUR	NO DRY EYE, DRY NOSE, DRY SKIN
NONPİTTİNG EDEMA	PİTTİNG EDEMA
BURNING IN URINE	URINARY INCONTINENCE
SLEEPING DISORDER	Ç TOO MUCH SLEEPING, HARD TO WAKE UP
HOT FLASH	CHİLL

NOT GAINING WEIGHT	INABILITY TO LOSE WEIGHT
HOT SWEATING	COLD SWEATING
NIGHT SWEATING	SPONTANEOUS SWEATING DAY AND NIGHT
THE PRESENCE OF A BAD SMELL	NO BAD SMELL
LOW AND YELLOW URINE	PLENTY OF LIGHT COLORED URINE
SOLID AND HARD STOOL	SOFT STOOL
COMPLAINTS INCREASE WITH DAYTIME OR HEAT APPLICATION	COMPLAINTS INCREASE WITH NIGHT AND COLD APPLICATION
COMPLAINTS INCREASE WITH MOVEMENT	COMPLAINTS INCREASE WITH REST
INCREASE OF COMPLAINTS IN HOT AND DRY WEATHER	INCREASE OF COMPLAINTS IN RAINY AND HUMID WEATHER

If a patient has dry mouth, prefers cold foods and desires to drink a lot of water, this indicates that the pool is hot. If there is a desire to drink less water and prefers hot foods, this indicates that the pool is cold. In some patients, hot pool symptoms and cold pool symptoms may occur together. For example, a patient may not want to drink much water even though he has a dry mouth. In other words, it tries to relieve dry mouth with a small amount of water. This condition is a typical symptom for phlegm. Phlegm is a type of damp. When it responds to dampness by increasing body temperature, it is called phlegm. You can also call this hot damp (Figure 35). The heat in the phlegm causes dry mouth, and the damp causes the person not to want to drink much water.

PHLEGM

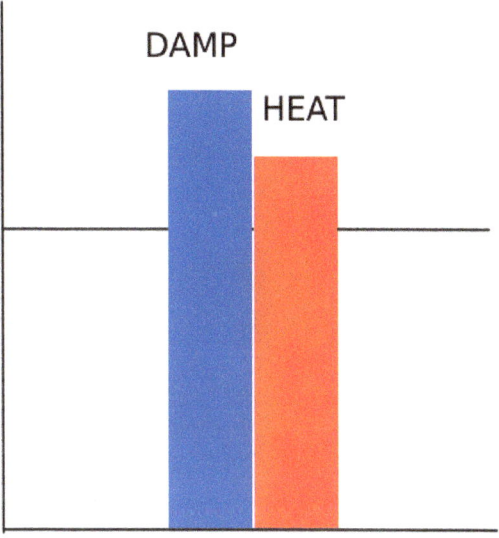

Figure 35: Phlegm

Dryness symptoms indicate that the pool is hot. In the presence of a hot pool where the cold water fountain flows insufficiently, dryness of the skin, nose or eyes may occur (Figure 36). If the dryness is in the nose or skin, the metal pool is considered hot, and if it is in the eyes, the wood pool is considered hot.

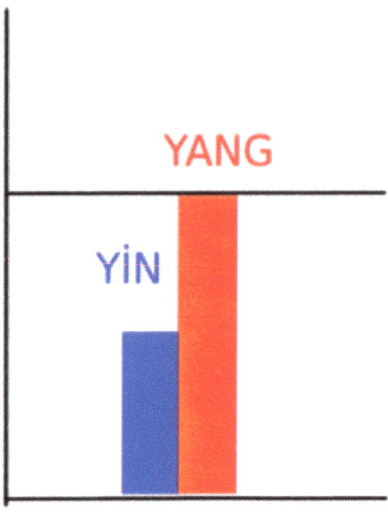

Figure 36: Yin deficiency

Although water retention and edema in the body seem to indicate a cold pool, they can sometimes occur in the presence of a hot pool (Figure 37). In cases where the pool is cold due to Yang deficiency, pitting edema occurs because the Yang energy required for the movement of the liquid is insufficient. There is a possibility of edema in the upper extremity in cases of insufficient lung Yang, in the lower extremity in cases of insufficient kidney Yang, and in both the upper and lower extremities in cases of insufficient spleen Yang. The edema that occurs in cases where the pool is hot due to yin deficiency is stiff and usually does not leave a pit. Just as the predominance of Yang causes tension in the pulse, edema where Yang is dominant also has a tense and hard structure.

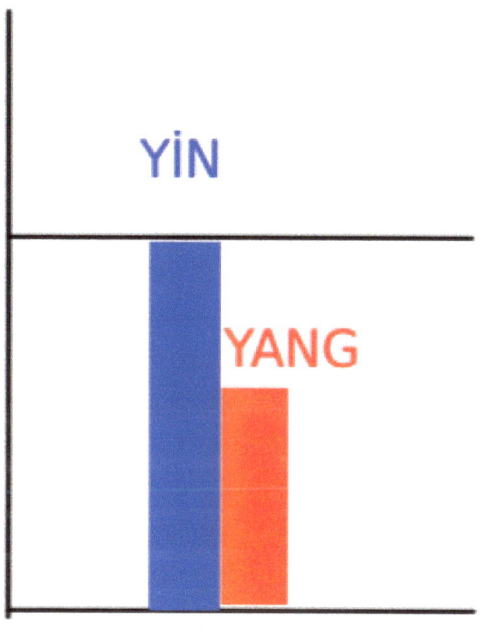

Figure 37: Yang deficiency

A wrong meaning may arise from the a contrario of the sentence "Dryness indicates that the pool is hot." In other words, if there is a runny nose and runny eyes, it does not mean that the pool is cold. Since discharge is a type of moisture, do not think that nasal and eye discharge indicates that the pool is cold. Nasal and eye discharge may be due to a hot pathogen or a damp pathogen. Cold discharge occurs in damp pathogens, and warm discharge occurs in warm pathogens. Since wind is the means by which external pathogens enter the body, you will see external pathogens written as "Wind hot" or "Wind cold" in the sources. Nasal and eye discharge can be observed in most cases caused by the wind hot pathogen. When the mucosal surfaces of the body that open to the outside are invaded by a "hot pathogen", if the body fluids are sufficient, this heat is tried to be balanced with the body fluids and this situation is reflected in the clinic as nasal discharge and eye discharge. Although the patient feels burning and dryness in the eyes and nose, there is discharge. The discharge may turn purulent in a short time. Similarly, in cases of gastroenteritis due to the Yang pathogen, diarrhea is observed in the patient. This diarrhea causes burning around the patient's anus and has a foul odor (Figure 38).

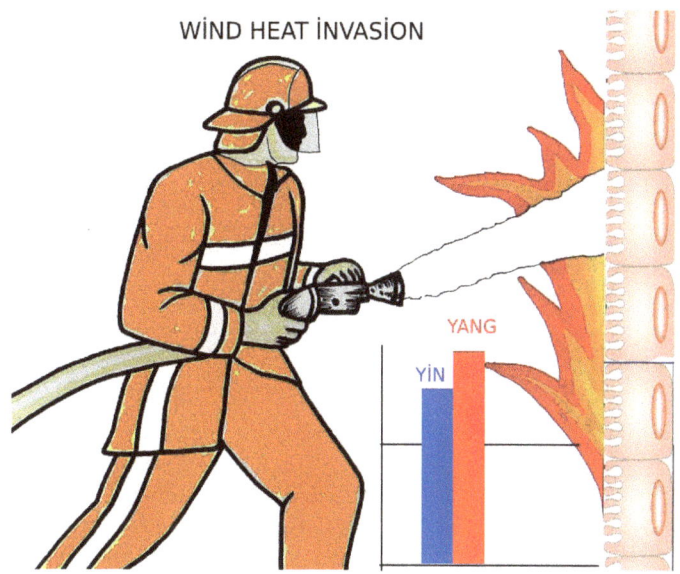

Figure 38: Pathogenesis of discharge in wind cold invasion

While noise and light belong to Yang, silence and darkness belong to Yin. For this reason, we will think that the pool is hot in cases of "noise and light aversion", which we see especially in migraine patients.

Inability to fall asleep or waking up frequently indicates that the pool is hot, while complaints of oversleeping and difficulty waking up in the morning indicate that the pool is cold. In cases where the cold water fountain flows insufficiently and the pool is hot due to Yin deficiency, sometimes the patient's relatives may mislead you. These patients want to complete their Yin through sleep. Especially if the patient is unemployed or retired, his/her relatives may tell you that the patient sleeps too much. However, when you question him, you get the story that the patient cannot sleep even if he lies down.

The hot flush symptom indicates that the pool is hot, while the chill symptom indicates that the pool is cold. I think it goes without saying that this sentence is valid for chronic deficiency cases. If the hot water fountain does not flow insufficiently, people will feel cold; if the cold water fountain does not flow insufficiently, they will experience hot flushes. This complaint, which we see frequently especially in post-menopausal patients, is mostly seen in cases where the kidney pool is hot, but it can also be seen in cases where other pools are hot. In cases of excess situation is different. In the early phase of excess cases when the Yin or Yang pathogen invades the body, that is, in the external phase when the pathogen settles between the skin and muscles, the patient becomes cold. One of the functions of "Wei Qi" located between the skin and the muscles is to warm the muscles underneath. When the external pathogen settles in this area where "Wei Qi" settles, this function of "Wei Qi" is blocked. For this reason, the patient feels cold whether it is a "cold pathogen" or a "hot pathogen". This chill is much more evident in the presence of a "cold pathogen". If you want to get more detailed information about this subject, you can look at the six-stage classification for cold pathogens and the four-level classification for hot pathogens.

We have mentioned the bad smell before. Just as food that is not refrigerated and left outside in the heat stinks, if there is a bad odor on the body, the pool is hot (Figure 39). This can be empty hot or full hot. If there is a strong odor in the stool, there is heat in the intestines, if there is a strong odor in the urine, there is heat in the bladder, if there is a strong odor in the armpit, there is heat in the heart or liver, and if there is a strong odor in the mouth, there is heat in the stomach. We said that bad breath may be due to lung and kidney heat as well as stomach heat.

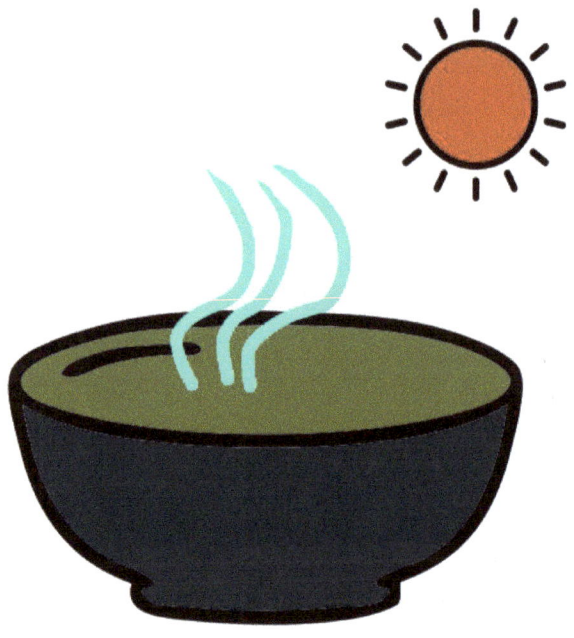

Figure 39: Image of food spoiling in heat

When the body temperature increases, it tries to cool itself by sweating. So, sweating is expected when the body is hot, which is called hot sweating. If the patient sweats only at night, this is typical for Yin deficiencies. If the cold water fountain flows insufficiently and the pool is therefore hot, why does the patient sweat only at night? Because sweat is also a body fluid and loss through sweat further reduces body fluid. For this reason, the patient does not sweat during the day, but it is at night when Yin is most intense. In some patients, sweating occurs even though the body is cold, which is called cold sweating. This occurs especially in lung Yang deficiency or lung Qi deficiency. While function belongs to Yang, structure belongs to Yin. One of the functions of the lung is to open and close sweat pores in the skin. The lungs, through "Wei Qi", open the pores when the body is hot and close them when it is cold. When the Yang or Qi of the lung is insufficient, the patient sweats constantly because the sweat pores remain open.

In patients who complain about not being able to gain weight, the pool is usually hot, while in patients who say they gain weight even if they drink water, the pool is usually cold.

A small amount of urine and a yellow color indicates that the pool is hot, and a large amount and a light color indicates that the pool is cold. Burning sensation while urinating indicates that the pool is hot, while urinary incontinence indicates that the pool is cold. You may hear from many post-menopausal patients that they have burning sensation, have a small amount of urine, and cannot hold their urine. So you may find that hot and cold pool symptoms occur together. In this case, you will think that the patient has kidney Yin and Yang deficiency together.

While solid and hard stool indicates that the metal pool is hot, soft stool indicates that it is cold. In cases where the cold water fountain opening into the metal pool has insufficient flow, the stool becomes dry and the patient has difficulty in defecating. In cases where the hot water fountain opening into the metal pool has insufficient flow, the stool is soft. But there is an issue that requires attention here. These patients may say they are constipated even though their stools are soft. Since Yang is insufficient, intestinal motility is low and the patient generally cannot defecate every day, but defecates every two to three days or once a week. But when you question him, he says his stool is soft.

Finally, let's close this discussion by touching on the last three symptoms in the table. If the complaints increase during the daytime, with heat application, movement or in hot and dry weather, it indicates that the pool is hot. If it increases at night, with cold application, at rest, or in cold and humid weather, it indicates that the pool is cold. This information applies specifically to musculoskeletal diseases, but not to all diseases. For example, in cases of tinnitus due to kidney Yin deficiency, tinnitus increases at night even though the pool is warm. Likewise, in people with cough due to lung Yin deficiency, the cough complaint increases at night, even though the pool is hot. These questions are very important in determining the type of musculoskeletal pain. If the patient's pain increases during the day, with heat application, movement, or in hot and dry weather, it is called Yang dominant pain. If the patient's pain increases at night, with cold application, at rest, or in cold and humid weather, it is called Yin dominant pain. As with every disease, distinguishing whether the pool is hot or cold will guide us in the treatment of musculoskeletal system pain. There is something I want to draw your attention to here. Although damp type pains are Yin dominant pains, they can sometimes be confused with Yang dominant pains. Damp type pains, like Yang dominant pains, increase when movement is started, there is a period of stiffness, and then they relax. You often see morning stiffness in these patients. The patient says that this pain decreases or disappears 1-2 hours after starting the movement. Therefore, if a patient says that his pain increases with movement, you need to examine this a little more. It should be clarified whether this pain, which increases with movement, continues to increase or decrease throughout the day. Another feature of damp-type pain is that the pain increases with pressure. For example, when a patient with damp-type hip pain lies on the side where the discomfort occurs, the pain increases. Even if a patient with damp-type shoulder pain puts a bag on his shoulder, his pain increases due to the pressure effect.

PHYSICAL EXAMINATION

Our second important parameter in evaluating whether the pool is hot or cold is physical examination. We also talked about smells and sounds in the general information section we gave about the five element theory. We said that a strong odor in a patient indicates that the pool is hot. We also said that a good doctor can make a diagnosis even if he hears a patient's voice from behind the door. If we ignore rarely used examination methods such as smelling and listening to the patient's voice, inspection and palpation are the two main methods we use in physical examination. We can include tongue examination in inspection and pulse examination in palpation.

INSPECTION AND TONGUE EXAMINATION

If the patient seems restless, the pool is usually warm. Patients we consider to be moody are more likely to be Yang dominant. Patients where the pool is cool usually appear calm.

Hyperemia indicates that the pool is hot. This hyperemia may occur in the eyes or tongue. Sometimes it can occur on the skin along a meridian course or without a meridian course. Paleness indicates a cold pool. This paleness may occur on the skin, tongue or lips. Edema observed without hyperemia in tissues and joints also indicates a cold pool. The dry and thin appearance of the skin indicates that the metal pool is hot, while the moist and thick appearance of the skin indicates that it is cold.

If the patient is thin, it indicates that the pool is hot, and if the patient is overweight, it indicates that it is cold. If you decide whether the pool is hot or cold based solely on the patient's weight, you will often make mistakes. There are many patients who are thin and the pool is cold, and patients who are overweight but the pool is hot.

We said that tongue examination is also a kind of inspection method. I will not talk about the tongue examination in detail here. In summary, hyperemia, dryness and cracking in the tongue body, yellowing of the tongue fur, and partial or complete loss of the tongue fur are hot pool findings. A normal tongue fur is a thin, white layer. Tongue fur reflects the condition of the Yang organs, especially the stomach. It gives us an idea about the nature of the external pathogen and the body's response to this pathogen. A pale tongue body, a swollen and moist appearance accompanied by tooth marks, and a thick and white tongue fur indicate a cold pool. The appearance of tongue fur changes very quickly with external factors. For this reason, acute excess cases should be evaluated more from the tongue fur, and chronic deficiency cases should be evaluated more from the tongue corpus.

In the light of this brief information, let's make an evaluation based on sample tongue images.

EXAMPLE 1:

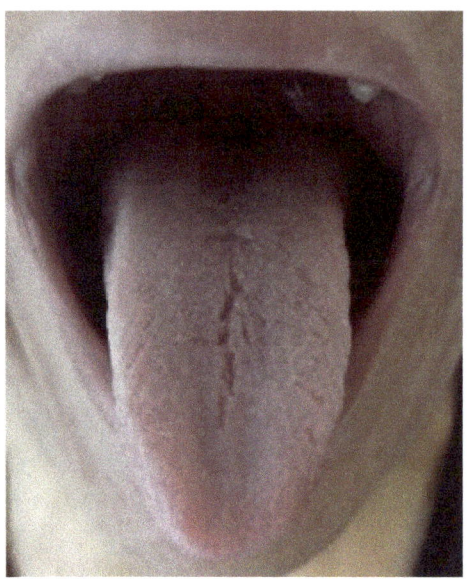

Figure 40: Sample tongue image

The tongue in Figure 40 looks dry, the tongue rust is missing, and there is a cleft in the middle of the tongue. The fact that the cleft is in the center of the tongue indicates a soil pool. In this case, we can say that the soil pool is hot. In other words, we can easily diagnose the patient with "Stomach Yin deficiency". Thus, we both found the faulty pool and commented on the temperature of the pool through the tongue (Figure 41).

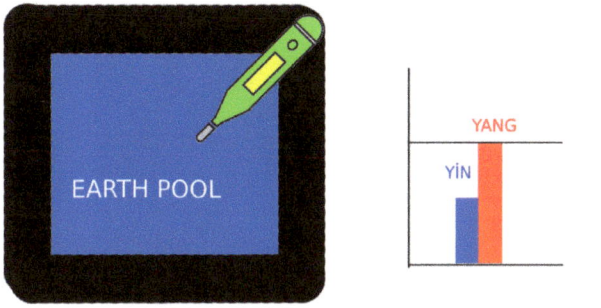

Figure 41: Stomach Yin deficiency

EXAMPLE 2:

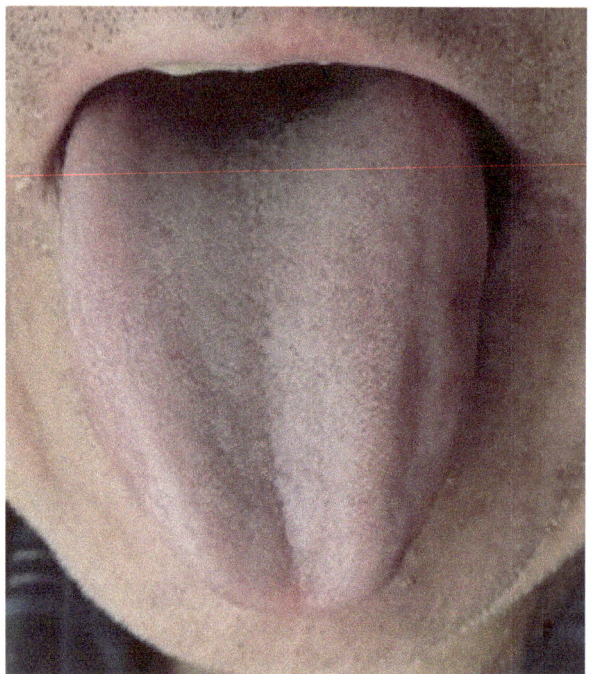

Figure 42: Sample tongue image

The body of the tongue in Figure 42 looks swollen, even though there are no tooth marks. Color is pale, tongue fur is white. These findings show us that the pool is cold. Since the spleen is the organ responsible for the transport of fluids, its deficiency usually results in a swollen appearance throughout the tongue. In other words, do not think that since the earth element is located in the center of the tongue, there will only be a swollen appearance in the center. In light of these findings, we can diagnose the patient with "Spleen Yang deficiency" (Figure 43). I think that the damp accumulated in this patient due to spleen deficiency tends to gradually turn into phlegm. Because if there was pure spleen Yang deficiency, the tongue corpus would appear moist. Here, the tongue has a slightly dry appearance.

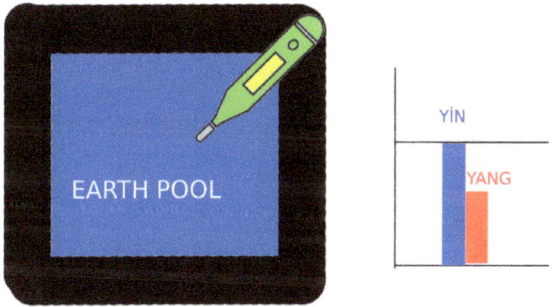

Figure 43: Spleen Yang deficiency

EXAMPLE 3:

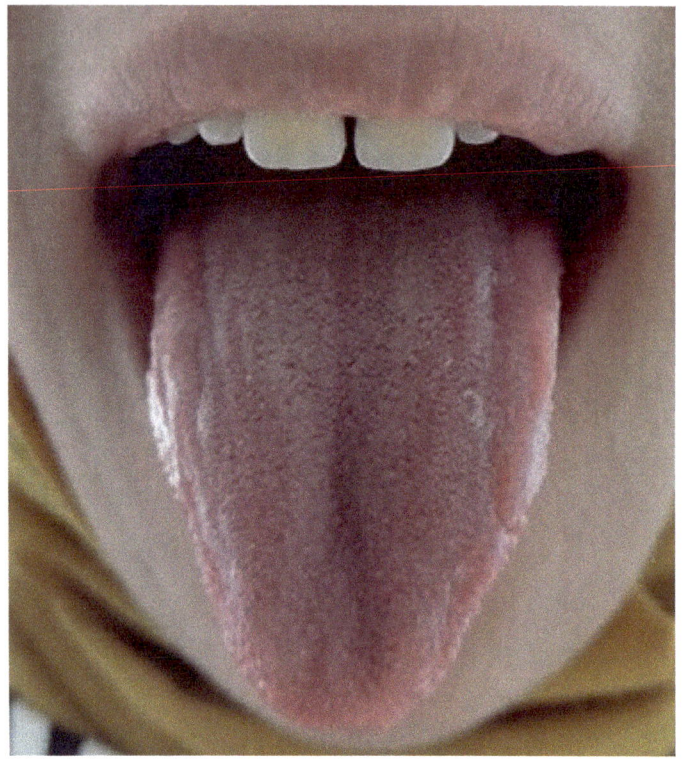

Figure 44: Sample tongue image

Although the tongue in Figure 44 does not appear very clearly in the photograph, a hyperemic appearance is observed along its lateral aspect and at the tip of the tongue. Hyperemia in the tongue corpus indicates that the pool is hot. The pool may be hot for two reasons. Either the hot water fountain is flowing too much or the cold water fountain is flowing insufficiently. So it is either due to excess or due to insufficiency. In order to say that the pool is warm due to Yin deficiency, there must be either a loss of tongue fur or a crack in the tongue corpus. Since there is no such appearance in this tongue, it was understood that the case was full hot and not empty hot. In this case, our definition is the full heat of the heart and liver (Figure 45).

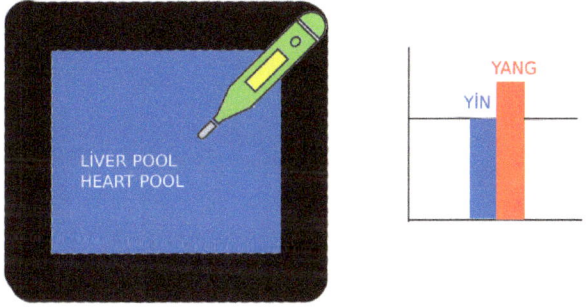

Figure 45: The full heat of the liver and heart pool

EXAMPLE 4:

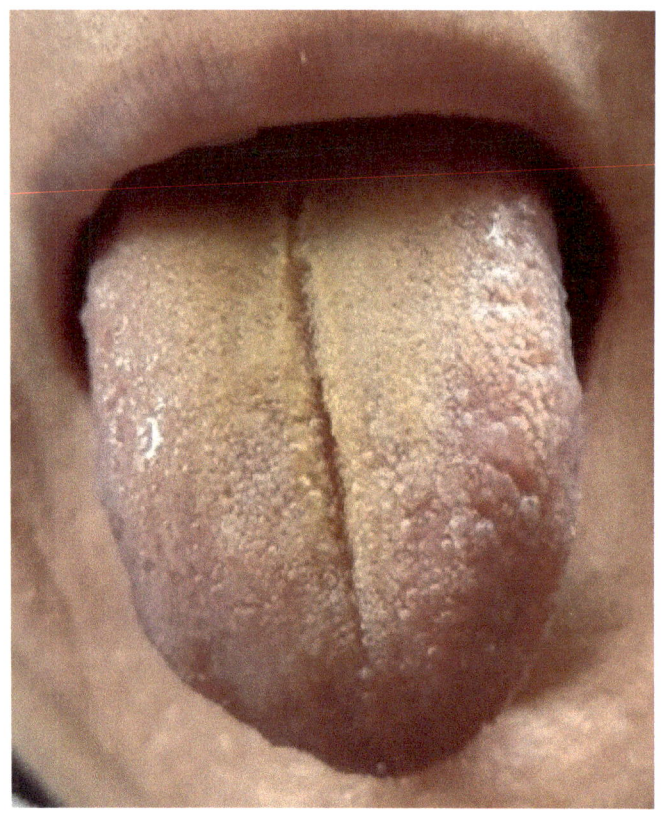

Figure46: Sample tongue image

The fact that there is a cleft in the tongue body from posterior to anterior in the figure 46 and the yellow color of the tongue fur indicates that the pool is hot. Such clefts in the midline extending to the anterior of the tongue are called "Heart clefts". This situation occurs in "Stomach and heart Yin deficiency". In Yin deficiencies, the tongue corpus is generally thin. This language corpus is not thin-looking. At the same time, although there is stomach Yin deficiency, there is no loss of tongue fur. On the contrary, there is some thickening and yellowing. Apparently, in this case, there is phlegm accumulation secondary to stomach Yin deficiency (Figure 47). In other words, the patient has both deficiency and excess. You will see such cases very often in the clinic, where deficiency and excess are combined.

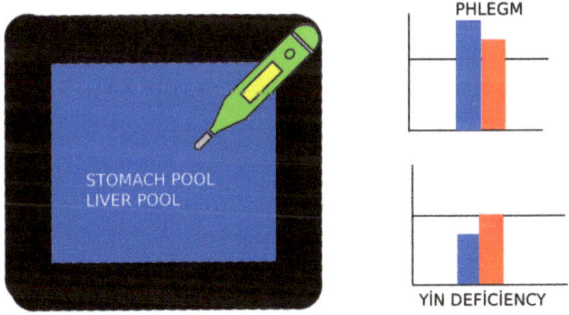

Figure 47: Heart and stomach Yin deficiency and phlegm

EXAMPLE 5:

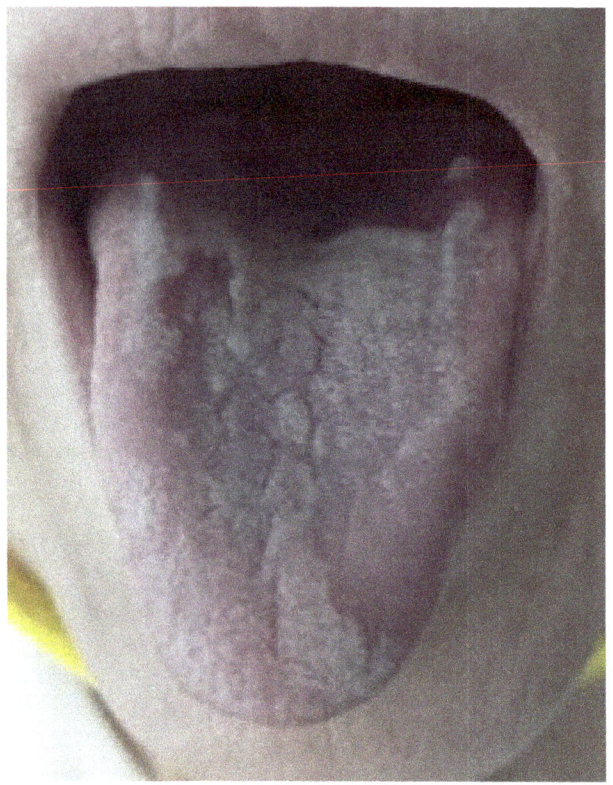

Figure 48: Sample tongue image

In the example tongue image in Figure 48, the tongue body is dry and there are cracks in some places. Tongue fur is white in color and losses are observed in some places. Loss of tongue fur, cracks in the tongue body and dryness indicate stomach Yin deficiency. Also, we can say that this patient's Yang level is probably low too. Because if Yang was very prominent, we would have seen hyperemia in the tongue corpus and yellowing of the tongue fur. In this case, it can be thought that stomach Yin and Yang deficiency is present together in the case, but stomach Yin deficiency is more prominent (Figure 49).

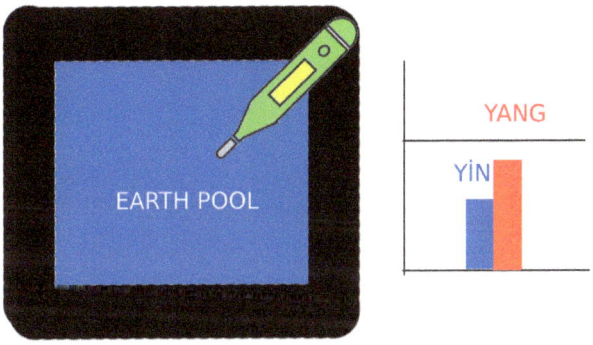

Figure 49: Yin-Yang deficiency, where Yin deficiency is more pronounced

EXAMPLE 6:

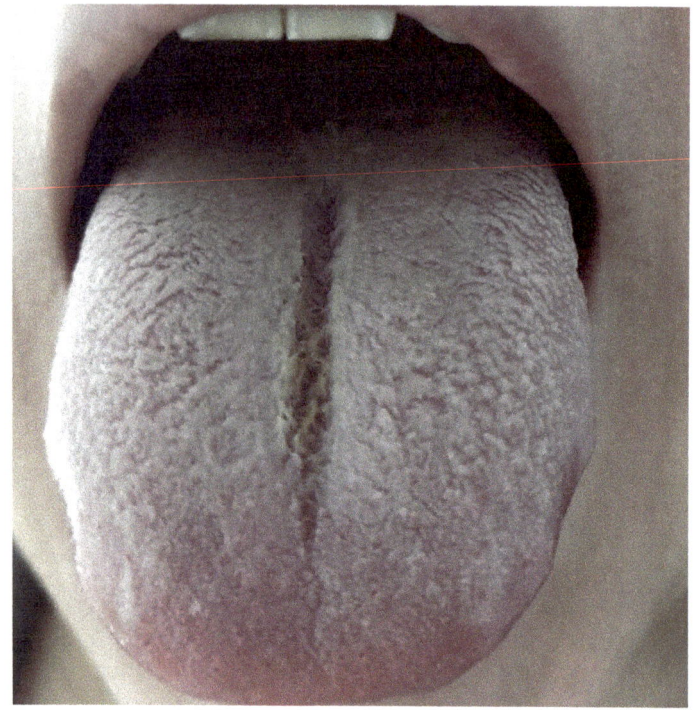

Figure 50: Sample tongue image

In the sample tongue image in Figure 50, the tongue body is observed as swollen. The tongue is observed to be partially hyperemic in the anterior part. Although the tongue fur is thick and white in color, it has started to turn partially yellow in the middle. The appearance of a crack in the middle of the tongue belongs to the tongue fur, not to the tongue corpus. These findings suggest that the dampness pathogen affects the earth pool. Tongue fur thickens in the presence of dampness pathogen. If the body responds to dampness by increasing its Yang, this dampness turns into phlegm. According to the five element theory, certain external pathogenic factors affect certain organs more. The dampness pathogen mostly affects the earth element. The slight hyperemia at the tip of the tongue suggests that the heat increase caused by damp in the earth element also spreads to the metal element, the son of the earth. This is a case of excess. Our diagnosis is phlegm secondary to moisture in the earth pool and "Full hot" caused by phlegm in the metal pool (Figure 51).

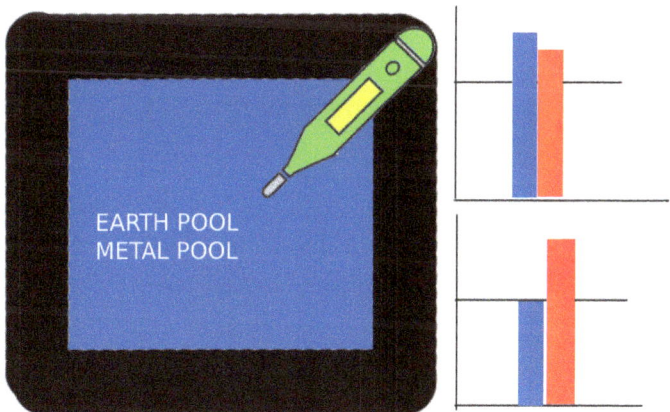

Figure 51: Phlegm in the earth pool, full hot in the metal pool

Let's end the inspection method we use to diagnose whether the faulty pool is hot or cold and continue with the palpation method.

PALPATION

To understand whether the faulty pool is hot or cold, put your hand into the pool and check its temperature, that is, touch the patient. Touching the patient's face, hand or even foot will give you an idea about most pools whose temperature you are curious about. The temperature of the patient's face gives an idea about the upper jiao, the temperature of the hands gives an idea about the upper and middle jiao, and the temperature of the feet gives an idea about the lower jiao. If a patient has a complaint about the course of the meridian, such as pain, check the temperature of the painful area with your hand. Even in organ disorders, the temperature may differ in the skin area around the location where the organ is located. For example, in patients with "Kidney Yang deficiency", when you touch the sides of the lumbar region, you can easily feel that it is colder than other areas.

PULSE EXAMINATION

Pulse examination, which is a palpation method, is an important form of examination that gives us an idea about whether the faulty pool is hot or cold. Pulse examination, which could constitute a volume of a book on its own, will not be discussed in detail; just like the tongue examination, I will try to simplify and explain it as I use it in the clinic. During the pulse examination, I recommend that you pay attention to four characteristics of the pulse. Strength, depth, thickness and speed of the pulse (Figure 52).

- IS THE PULSE STRONG OR WEAK?
- SUPERFICIAL OR DEEP?
- THIN OR THICK?
- FAST OR SLOW?

Figure 52: Four qualities of the pulse

As the pool warms up, the pulse becomes shallower. So, in patients whose pulse we see superficially, we will say that the pool is hot. The fact that the pool is hot may be due to the excessive flow of the hot water fountain, or it may be due to the insufficient flow of the cold water fountain. In other words, the case may be a case of excess or a case of deficiency. If the pool is hot due to excessive flow from the hot water fountain, the pulse will be both shallow and strong. If the pool is hot due to insufficient flow from the cold water fountain, the pulse is superficial but weak. When it comes to superficial pulse, the human mind can perceive it as a strong pulse. This kind of thinking is wrong. So, if a superficial pulse does not disappear when you press it, it is strong and is due to excess; if it disappears immediately when you press it, it is weak and is due to deciency. As the pool cools, the pulse deepens. Let's make the same sentence for the cold pool as we did for the hot pool. The coldness of the pool may be due to the excessive flow of the cold water fountain, or it may be due to the insufficient flow of the hot water fountain. In other words, the case may be a case of excess or a case of deficiency. If the pool is cold due to excessive flow from the cold water fountain, the pulse will be both deep and strong. If the pool is cold due to insufficient flow of the hot water fountain, the pulse is deep and weak. (Figure 53).

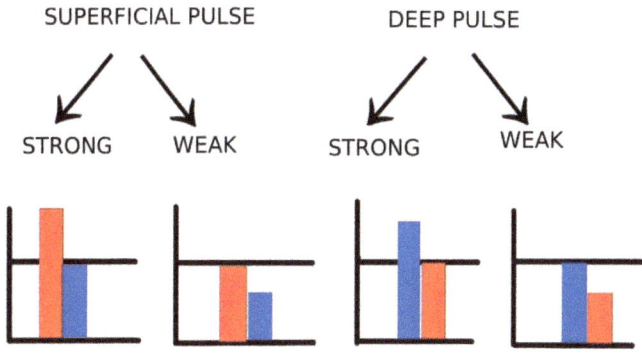

Figure 53: Types of superficial and deep pulses

Here, let's not forget to mention an exception related to environmental pathogenic factors. When the environmental cold pathogen enters the body, it settles between the skin and muscles in the early stage, which is called the external stage. If the disease cannot be eradicated at this stage, it passes to the internal stage. When the cold pathogen is in the external stage, the pulse is superficial. It deepens when it passes into the internal phase. Then we will keep in mind this exceptional case of the pulse in infectious diseases. In the external phases of both "Hot" and "Cold" external pathogenic factors, the pulse is superficial.

Let's come to the thickness of the pulse. Let's simplify the issue this way. Since blood consists of plasma and blood cells, the less plasma in the blood, the thinner the pulse. In other words, a thin pulse is an indication of Yin deficiency or dryness. It is "Yang" that gives tension to the pulse. In this case, in a patient with Yin deficiency, if Yang is also inadequate, the pulse will be both thin and loose, like cotton thread. If Yin is deficient but Yang is normal or excessive, the pulse will be thin and tense, like a guitar string. If the pulse feels thick, you can imagine that the plasma portion of the blood is excessive. So a thick pulse indicates the presence of moisture (Figure 54).

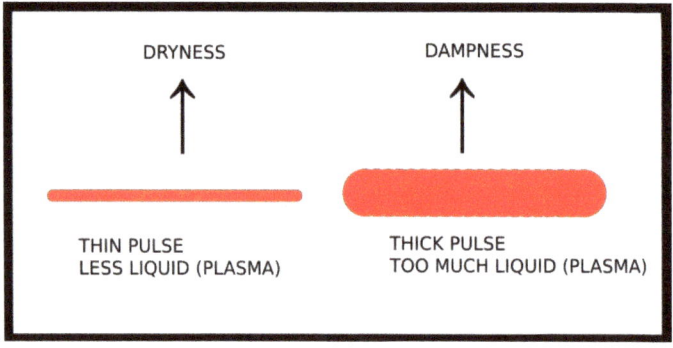

Figure 54: Thickness of the pulse

If the pulse feels thick but its consistency is soft, it means that the body did not respond to the dampness pathogen by increasing its Yang. In other words, this indicates the presence of pure dampness. If the pulse feels thick but has a hard consistency, then the body has responded to the

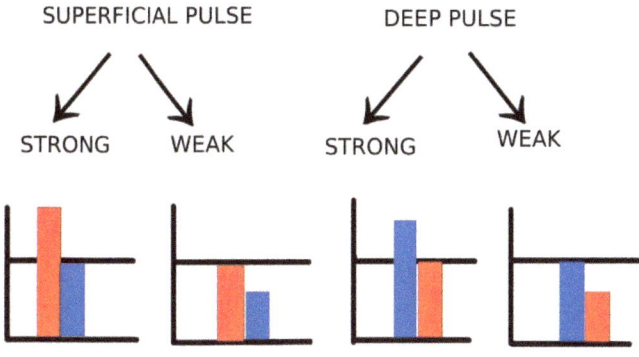

Figure 53: Types of superficial and deep pulses

Here, let's not forget to mention an exception related to environmental pathogenic factors. When the environmental cold pathogen enters the body, it settles between the skin and muscles in the early stage, which is called the external stage. If the disease cannot be eradicated at this stage, it passes to the internal stage. When the cold pathogen is in the external stage, the pulse is superficial. It deepens when it passes into the internal phase. Then we will keep in mind this exceptional case of the pulse in infectious diseases. In the external phases of both "Hot" and "Cold" external pathogenic factors, the pulse is superficial.

Let's come to the thickness of the pulse. Let's simplify the issue this way. Since blood consists of plasma and blood cells, the less plasma in the blood, the thinner the pulse. In other words, a thin pulse is an indication of Yin deficiency or dryness. It is "Yang" that gives tension to the pulse. In this case, in a patient with Yin deficiency, if Yang is also inadequate, the pulse will be both thin and loose, like cotton thread. If Yin is deficient but Yang is normal or excessive, the pulse will be thin and tense, like a guitar string. If the pulse feels thick, you can imagine that the plasma portion of the blood is excessive. So a thick pulse indicates the presence of moisture (Figure 54).

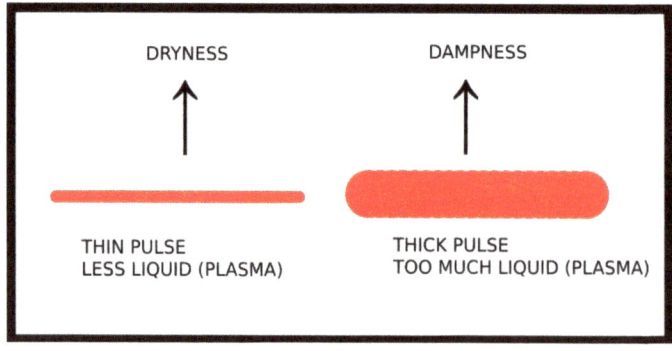

Figure 54: Thickness of the pulse

If the pulse feels thick but its consistency is soft, it means that the body did not respond to the dampness pathogen by increasing its Yang. In other words, this indicates the presence of pure dampness. If the pulse feels thick but has a hard consistency, then the body has responded to the dampness pathogen by increasing its Yang, which is called slippery pulse (Figure 55). The slippery pulse felt in the presence of phlegm is described as if there was a pearl under the finger.

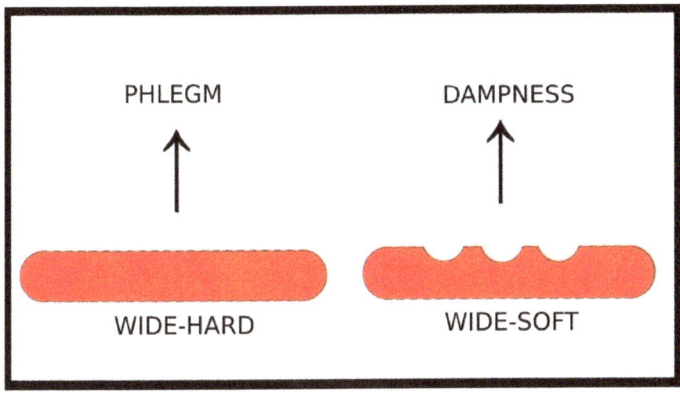

Figure 55: Slippery pulse

Although the pulse rate changes with age, roughly below 60 beats per minute is considered low, and above 80 beats per minute is considered rapid. Heart rate actually indicates the state of the heart pool. Although it is written in the sources that the heart rate increases when Yang is dominant in any organ, the heart rate actually increases if the organ with increased Yang affects the heart through one of the mother-son or grandmother-grandson interactions. Then, if the heart rate is above 80 beats per minute, we will say that the heart pool is hot, and if it is below 60, we will say that the heart pool is cold (Figure 56).

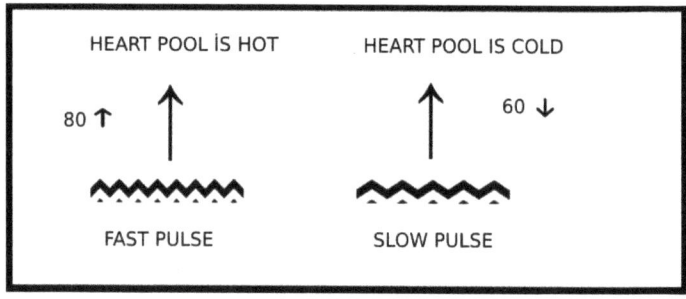

Figure 56: Heart rate

AUTHORS' COMMENT

Since we physicians, trained in Modern Medicine, generally interpret diseases diagnosed with Western Medicine according to TCM, it is natural for us to benefit from authorial comments about the temperature of the pool we find. For example, depression is often considered a disease of the upper jiao. According to the five element theory, joy is the emotion associated with the heart and sadness is the emotion associated with the lungs. If depression is interpreted as the patient's lack of joy and sadness, it will be better understood why the faulty pool is the heart and lungs located in the upper jiao. In depression, the liver pool is often mentioned among the faulty pools too. While some authors only nourish Yin in the treatment of depression, others nourish Yang as well. As can be seen, just as there are disagreements among the authorities in finding the faulty pool, there can also be disagreements about the temperature of the pool. If we are as aware of these controversies as possible, we will have the opportunity to interpret diseases from different perspectives.

THİRD STEP

EDIT THE TEMPERATURE OF THE FAULTY POOL

In the first step, we found the faulty pool. In the second step, we checked the temperature of the faulty pool. In the third step, we will regulate the temperature of the pool using hot and cold water fountains opening into the pool (Figure 57). If Yang energy is deficient in an organ, the process of increasing Yang energy is called Yang tonification. We will call this "Turning on the hot water fountain." If Yin energy is deficient in an organ, the process of increasing Yin energy is called Yin tonification. We will call this "Turning on the cold water fountain." If Yang energy is excessive in an organ, the process of reducing Yang energy is called Yang sedation. We will call this "Turning off the hot water fountain". If Yin energy is excessive in an organ, the process of reducing Yin energy is called Yin sedation. We will call this "Turning off the cold water fountain".

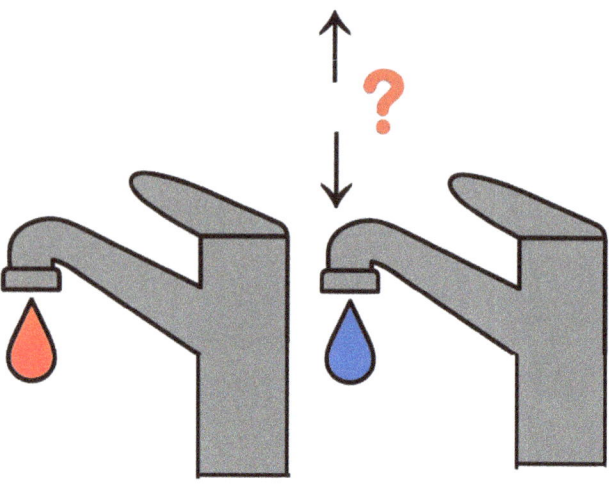

Figure 57: Process of regulating the temperature of the faulty pool

Will we balance the temperature of the cold pool by opening the hot water tap or closing the cold water tap? Will we balance the temperature of the hot pool by opening the cold water tap or closing the hot water tap?

Let's answer these questions using the figure below (Figure 58). I got this shape from Thambirajah. I also explained it to you in my book titled "Systematic Acupuncture". I think this figure is very important for understanding the subject.

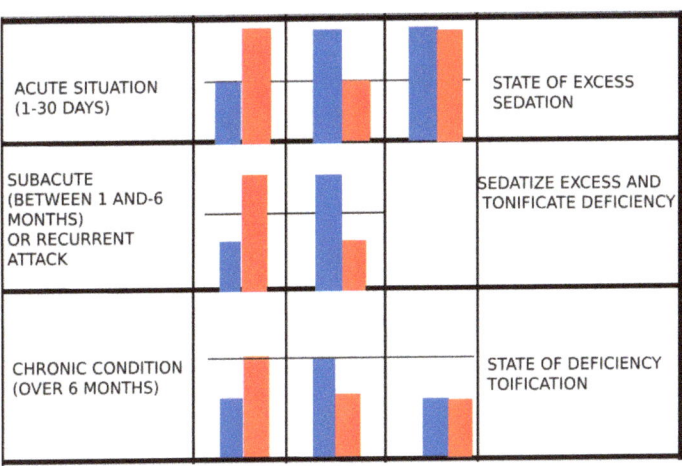

Figure 58: Procedure to be followed in cases of excess and deficiency

Cases of excess are treated by turning down the tap, while cases of deficiency are treated by opening the tap. In other words, sedation is performed in cases of excess and tonification is performed in cases of deficiency. Deciding whether the disease is a case of excess or deficiency is not easy for friends who are new to acupuncture training. As you gain experience in the tongue and pulse examination we have described, it will become much easier to make this decision. Friends who have not yet gained sufficient experience can make this decision by questioning the beginning of the patient's complaint. If the patient describes a complaint period of at most 30 days, the case is called an acute case or an excess case and is treated by turning off the taps. If the pool is hot, the hot water tap is closed; if the pool is cold, the cold water tap is closed. If cold pool symptoms and signs occur together with hot pool symptoms and signs, both taps are closed. If the patient indicates a period between 1 and 6 months for his complaint, the case is called subacute. In subacute cases, deficiency and excess are considered to occur together. Therefore, one of the taps is closed and the other is opened. If the pool is hot, the hot water tap is closed and the cold water tap is opened. If the pool is cold, the cold water tap is closed and the hot water tap is opened. If the patient describes his complaint as lasting longer than 6 months, it is called a chronic or deficiency case and is treated by opening the taps. If the pool is hot, the cold water tap is opened; if the pool is cold, the hot water tap is opened. In some cases of deficiency, findings indicating that the pool is hot may be accompanied by findings indicating that it is cold, or there may be no findings indicating that the pool is cold or hot. In this case, both taps are opened.

The Yin Yang diagram of recurrent chronic diseases such as asthma and migraine, which progress with occasional attacks, is just like the Yin Yang diagram of subacute diseases. Therefore, even if the disease is chronic, one tap is turned off and the other is opened during an attack.

It may not always be correct to decide on excess or deficiency based on the onset of the patient's complaint. Some cases with a chronic basis may present acutely to the clinic. For example, we would be wrong if we evaluated a patient with myocardial infarction as an acute case based on the beginning of his complaint. Just as we witness only the moment of an overflowing coffee pot, and we know that there is a warming phase before that overflow, we will know that some diseases that appear acute in the clinic may also develop on a chronic basis. For this reason, although there are some handicaps in diagnosing excess and deficiency based on the initial time of the patient's complaint, it will help you make the right decision in most cases.

Let's make what we said more understandable through an example case. Let's imagine a febrile case of gastroenteritis. Let's say their complaints started 2 days ago. We looked at his tongue and saw a yellow tongue fur. We felt the pulse as strong and superficial on the right side in the anterior position. In light of the symptoms and findings, we said that our faulty pool is the large intestine. Examination findings indicated that the pool was hot. We thought that the case was a case of excess, both from the duration of the complaints and the examination findings. Since the large intestine belongs to the metal element, it will be enough to turn off the hot water fountain that opens to the metal pool. The hot water fountain opening to the metal pool is the large intestine meridian. We will explain in the following passages how to turn off the tap on the large intestine meridian. For now, just understanding the logic of the approach will be enough. A question may come to mind: Can't we cool the hot metal pool by turning on the cold water fountain? We said that cases of excess are sedated and cases of deficiency are tonified. The process of opening the tap is the tonification process. In this case, the first thing we need to do is turn off the hot water tap. However, cooling the pool by turning on the cold water tap is also an alternative. If you do both operations at the same time, that is, if you turn off the hot water tap and open the cold water tap at the same time, the case may turn into a cold pool in a short time. In other words, although the patient's fever drops rapidly, cold diarrhea may occur. In hot diarrhea, the patient's stool smells very bad and causes a burning sensation around the anus. In cold diarrhea, the bad smell of the patient's stool and the burning sensation around the anus disappear, but the diarrhea continues. For this reason, it is beneficial not to continue the process of closing the hot water tap and opening the cold water tap for a long time, but to end it after 1-2 sessions. Even in cases where you only perform sedation, I recommend that you end the acupuncture sessions when the patient's complaint disappears.

Let our second example be a migraine patient. The patient says that the pain is sometimes in the temples, sometimes in the skull, and sometimes behind the eyes. The patient, who has had occasional attacks for 3 years, is disturbed by light and sound when he has pain, and is occasionally accompanied by nausea and vomiting. We could not see any significant feature in the patient's tongue examination, and we found the pulse to be superficial and weak in the left side guan area. In this patient, we thought the faulty pool was the gallbladder. From the symptoms and signs, we decided that the pool was hot. The case is a case of chronic deficiency and the pool is hot. If the patient comes to us at a time when he has no pain, it will be enough to turn on the cold water fountain leading to the wood pool. If it comes to us during an attack, we turn on the cold water fountain. If the pain is relieved, there is no need to do anything additional. If the pain is not relieved, we also turn off the hot water fountain.

Let's say a few more words about chronic cases and end the "third step". In my clinical practice I have found that the Yin Yang diagram in chronic cases may differ slightly from that shown in the figure above. For example, in cases of Yin deficiency, although Yin decreases, Yang may also partially decrease. In cases of Yang deficiency, although Yang decreases, Yin may also partially decrease. In other words, in chronic cases, the hot and cold pool Yin Yang diagram may look like the figure below (Figure 59).

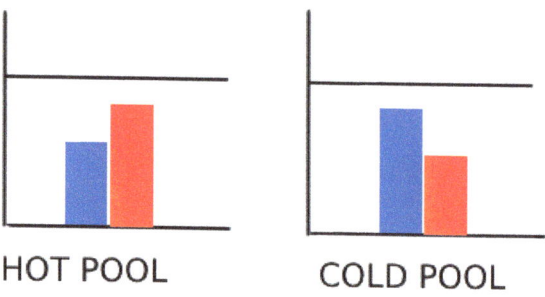

Figure 59: Yin Yang diagram in chronic cases

Let's give the case of chronic recurrent gastritis as an example to better understand what I am talking about. During the pain-free period of these patients, their Yin is very low, but their Yang is also partially low. During the attack, Yin cannot control Yang and Yang rises above normal. After the attack, it returns to its previous state (Figure 60).

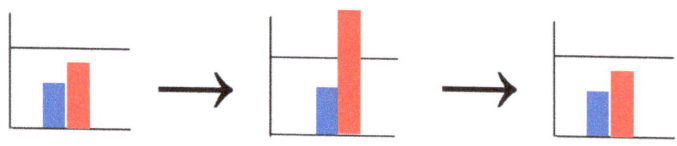

Figure 60: Yin Yang diagram in chronic recurrent gastritis

In these patients, if only the cold water fountain is turned on during the pain-free period and the hot water fountain is turned off for a long time during the attack period, the case usually turns into a cold pool. In this case, the patient starts to say that if I drink water, I feel swollen. So, what strategy should we follow in this case? If the patient is relieved by simply turning on the cold water fountain during the attack, there is no need to do anything additional. If it does not provide relief, the hot water fountain should be turned off for a short time, perhaps for 1 session. During the pain-free period, 2 or 3 cold water fountains and 1 hot water fountain should be turned on. You can apply this approach in all cases of chronic deficiency. In other words, in cases of deficiency where the pool is hot, it would be better if 1 hot water fountain is opened in addition to 2-3 cold water fountains. In cases of deficiency where the pool is cold, it would be better if 1 cold water fountain is opened in addition to 2-3 hot water fountains. In cases of deficiency where the pool is neither hot nor cold, it would be better to open 1 hot water tap and 1 cold water tap (Figure 61).

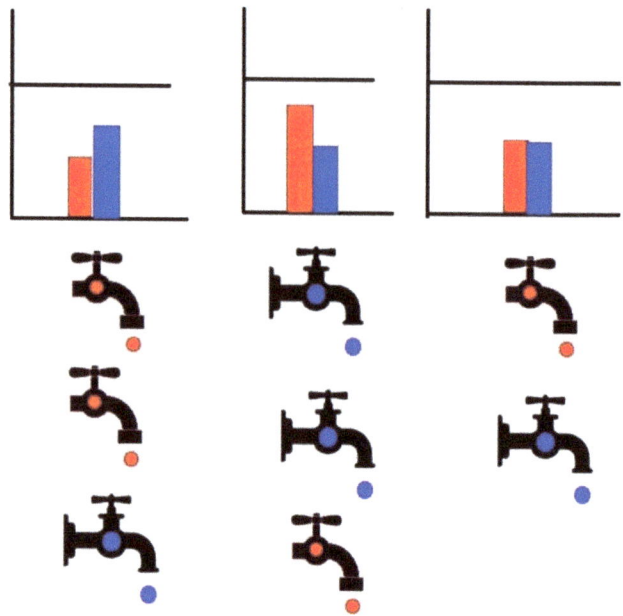

Figure 61: The treatment we recommend in cases of deficiency

As we partially mentioned in the language examination, you can also see that deficiency and excess occur together in many patients in the clinic. Phlegm cases due to spleen deficiency are examples of this, which we encounter very frequently in the clinic. In such a case, will we perform "Tonification" due to deficiency or "Sedation" due to excess? To make this decision, the patient's pulse is checked. If the pulse is weak, "Tonification" is performed, and if the pulse is strong, "Sedation" is performed.

Finally, let's end this passage by saying this. In the clinic, you may see many patients whose symptoms and signs simultaneously point to different pools. While summer may be dominant in one geography in the universe, winter may be dominant in another geography, and some of the faulty pools we find may be hot and some may be cold. Therefore, it is necessary to evaluate the temperature of each pool separately and treat it accordingly.

Thus, we learned how to approach diseases in "three steps". While explaining the "three steps", we did not mention how to use five element acupuncture in treatment, although we used the five element theory in the diagnosis part. From now on, I will explain how we use five element acupuncture in treatment. But before moving on to the subject, let us say a few additional words to complete what has been said so far. A student who reads reference books that approach diseases by defining "disease pattern according to internal organs" can say: Teacher, after what you have explained, I can now better understand the terms "Yin deficiency", "Yang deficiency", "Yin excess", "Yang excess" in these reference books. However, terms such as "Qi deficiency" and "Blood deficiency" are also used in these books. How should I understand these?

I can briefly answer this question as follows: If you do not have clear evidence that the pool is hot or cold, if you cannot say the pool is cold or hot, you can say Qi deficiency. Maybe some existing evidence might make the pool feel cold, but there is no evidence to support this. You can think of these cases as cases where Yin and Yang decrease together. For example, you evaluated a patient with chronic cough, hoarseness, and shortness of breath. You found the faulty pool to be a lung pool. To comment on the temperature of the pool, you examined the tongue and pulse. Although the pale and moist appearance of the tongue would suggest that the pool was cold, you did not find any additional evidence that the pool was cold. In this case, you can call the case lung Qi deficiency. During the treatment, you use the hot and cold water fountains leading to the metal pool in a balanced manner. So, if you open 1 hot water fountain, you also open 1 cold water fountain. Or if you are opening 2 hot water fountains, you also open 2 cold water fountains.

In cases of blood deficiency, the pool may be hot or cold. Blood is Yin in that it moisturizes and nourishes the tissues, and it is Yang in that it warms and moves the tissues. Tongue findings are typical in blood deficiencies. The tongue body is pale and thin. In Yang or Qi deficiencies, the tongue body is pale but swollen. In both Qi deficiencies and blood deficiencies where the pool is balmy, the pulse is as thin and soft as cotton thread. In cases where you have diagnosed blood deficiency, if the pool is cold, you turn on 2-3 hot water fountains and 1 cold water fountain. If the pool is hot, you turn on 2-3 cold water fountains and 1 hot water fountain. If the pool is balmy, you turn on 1-2 hot water fountains and 1-2 cold water fountains.

After this short additional information, I hope you will understand it much more easily when you read the source books that approach diseases by defining "disease patterns according to internal organs".

FIVE ELEMENT ACUPUNCTURE

Each meridian has points that balance the energy, which we call five shu (transport) points, located between the elbows and fingers or between the knees and toes (Table 3). The process of regulating the energy imbalance that occurs in the pool with the five shu points is called five element acupuncture. When you learn this treatment logic, you will be able to decide for yourself at which points you should open and close the hot and cold water taps filling the pool for each disease.

Table 3: Five shu points

Yin Meridians	Jing-Well (Wood)	Ying-Spring (Fire)	Shu-Stream (Earth)	Jing-River (Metal)	He-Sea (Water)
Lung	LU 11	LU 10	LU 9	LU 8	LU 5
Pericardium	PC 9	PC 8	PC 7	PC 5	PC 3
Heart	HT 9	HT 8	HT 7	HT 4	HT 3
Spleen	SP 1	SP 2	SP 3	SP 5	SP 9
Liver	LIV 1	LIV 2	LIV 3	LIV 4	LIV 8
Kidney	KID 1	KID 2	KID 3	KID 7	KID 10
Yang Meridians	Jing-Well (Metal)	Ying-Spring (Water)	Shu-Stream (Wood)	Jing-River (Fire)	He-Sea (Earth)
Large intestine	LI 1	LI 2	LI 3	LI 5	LI 11
Sanjiao	Sj 1	Sj 2	Sj 3	Sj 6	Sj 10
Small intestine	SI 1	SI 2	SI 3	SI 5	SI 8
Stomach	ST 45	ST 44	ST 43	ST 41	ST 36
Gall bladder	GB 44	GB 43	GB 41	GB 38	GB 34
Urine bladder	UB 67	UB 66	UB 65	UB 60	UB 40

In the table you see five shu points. These points start from the tips of the fingers and toes and end at the elbow and knee. As you can see, some of these points start with the number 1, while others start with different numbers. This is because there are points at the fingertips where the meridians either end or begin. If the meridians start from the fingertip, they start with the number 1. Each meridian ending at the fingertip ends with a different number. Therefore, you need to know which meridians start from the fingertip, which meridians end at the fingertip, and which number they end with.

The five shu points, starting from the fingertip and ending at the elbow and knee, are likened to a source of water coming out of a well and flowing into a spring, then into a stream, then into a river, then into the sea. For this reason, these points are named as well, spring, stream, river and sea points, starting from the distal end. In reference books, their Chinese and English expressions are usually given together (Table 4).

Table 4: Names of the five shu points

WELL POINT	JING-WELL
SPRING POINT	YING-SPRING
SRTEAM POINT	SHU-STREAM
RIVER POINT	JING-RIVER
SEA POINT	HE-SEA

In the system I plan to explain to you in a simplified way, the above nomenclature doesn't really matter. I've only included this nomenclature so that when you hear a sentence like "Well points or jing-well points are bled" in the source books, you understand that the first shu point on the fingertip is meant, or the fifth shu point is meant when it says sea points are pricked.

In order to memorize the five shu points more easily, let me look at the table from a bird's eye view and give you a few tips. The first three points go sequentially from the fingertip towards the proximal. The gallbladder is an exception. In the gallbladder, the first two points follow the order. The fourth point on the lung and liver meridians also follows the order. On other meridians, the fourth point does not follow the order. The fourth point is located near the hand and ankle, while the fifth point is located around the knee and elbow. What I said may seem confusing to the reader. It will be more clearly understood when we explain the points one by one in detail.

In the Yin meridians, we will name the points with the elements of wood, fire, earth, metal and water, respectively, starting from the fingertip. This nomenclature is important in the system we will explain. To make it easier to remember this sequence, imagine a view like this. There is a tree in front of you. The tree is planted in a metal flowerpot. The rays of the sun settling between the soil and the tree catch your eye, and water has leaked out of the metal pot (Figure 62).

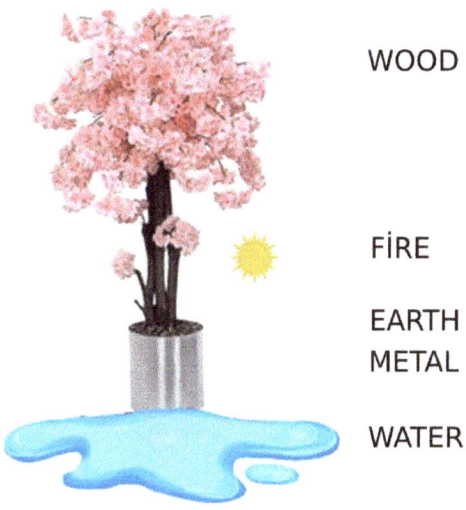

Figure 62: Naming order of the five shu points on the yin meridians

There are many different forms of five-element acupuncture applied in practice. Let's talk about them first so that the reader is aware of the different application methods of five element acupuncture.

In one form of five element acupuncture, the first two shu points, the well and spring points, are used for diseases related to the meridian course, while the last point, the sea point, is used for diseases of the organs. For example, the first two shu points of the stomach meridian (St 45, St 44) are used for diseases related to the meridian course such as frontal headache, while the sea point (St 36) is used for organ-related diseases such as gastritis. For diseases related to the esophagus, intermediate points are used. Since the Five Elements are associated with the five seasons, there is also a school that uses the five shu points depending on the season in which the symptoms appear. For example, if respiratory disease occurs in spring, the Lung's tree point (Lu 11) is used; if symptoms occur in winter, the Lung's Water point (Lu 5) is used. It is not a very useful method.

In another form of application of five element acupuncture, the tree points are used with a sedating maneuver to drive away the wind and a tonifying maneuver to increase the mobility of the organs. Fire points are used with a sedating maneuver to drive away fire and a tonifying maneuver to increase fire. Earth point is used with tonifying maneuver to increase nutrition and humidity and with sedating maneuver to decrease humidity. The metal point is used with a tonifying maneuver to increase dryness and a sedating maneuver to decrease dryness. Increasing dryness means encouraging perspiration. So tonification of the metal point is used to promote sweating, while sedation is used to reduce sweating. The water point is used with a tonifying maneuver to increase cold and a sedating maneuver to decrease cold.

The five element acupuncture styles I will teach you in the book will be different from the five element acupuncture practices I have described above. I plan to convey it to you as Radha Thambirajah conveyed it and as I have been using it for years and have personally observed its effectiveness.

FIVE SHU POINTS OF THE LUNG MERIDIAN

The lung meridian starts from the thorax and ends at the tip of the thumb. The point where it ends at the fingertip is the Lu 11 point. First, let's write the numbers of the five shu points on the meridian. We said that the lungs follow the order. The first four points will go in order (Lu11, Lu10, Lu9, Lu8). Fifth point does not fit in order (Lu 5). Here, the fifth point, that is, the Lu 5 point, is memorization. Now let's name these points one by one. We named Lu 11 wood, Lu 10 fire, Lu 9 earth, Lu 8 metal, and Lu 5 water (Figure 63).

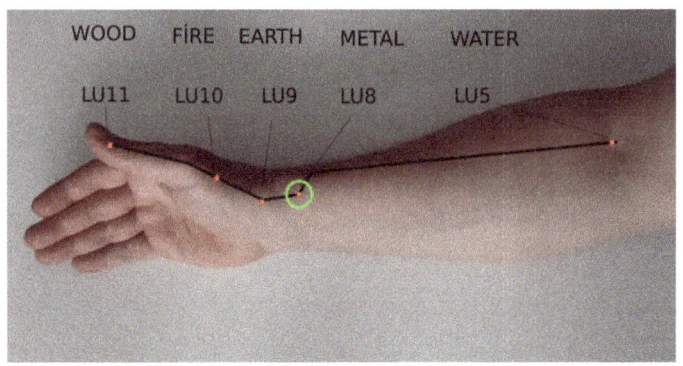

Figure 63: Five shu points of the lung meridian

In order to define these points, the first point we need to find on the meridian is the element point. Since the lung belongs to the metal element, the Lu 8 point, which is the metal point on the lung meridian, becomes the element point of the meridian. The point before the element point is the mother point or tonification point. The tonification point is the point that opens the tap. It feeds mostly Yin energy in Yin meridians, and mostly Yang energy in Yang meridians. Thambirajah puts this ratio as 90:10. However, if we remember that the Yin energy ratios in all Yin meridians and the Yang energy ratios in all Yang meridians are not the same, I believe that it would not be correct to say a sharply circumscribed ratio such as 90:10. Then, rather than specifying a sharply circumscribed ratio such as the tonification point nourishes 90% Yin and 10% Yang in the Yin meridians, it would be more accurate to say that it largely nourishes Yang and partly nourishes Yin. Likewise, the tonification point of the Yang meridians will feed largely Yang and partially Yin. In this case, the Lu 9 point before the element point on the lung meridian becomes the tonification point. The point before the tonification point is the grandmother point. The grandmother point increases Yang in Yin meridians; It increases Yin in Yang meridians. In other words, by activating the controlling interaction, draws the energy from the grandmother organ. Remember that in the controlling interaction, there is a transfer of energy from the Yin organ to the Yang organ, and from the Yang organ to the Yin organ. Therefore, the Lu 10 point on the lung meridian becomes the grandmother point. Think of the grandmother point on the Yin meridians as a hot water valve, and the grandmother point on the Yang meridians as a cold water valve (Figure 64).

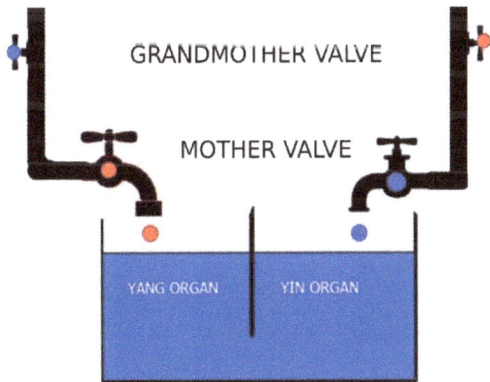

Figure 64: Representation of the nene point on the meridians

The next point after the element point is called the son point or sedation point. The point after the sedation point is the grandchild point. The son and grandson point sedates largely Yin in Yin meridians and largely Yang in Yang meridians. So you can think of the son and grandchild points as points that turn off the tap. In this case, the Lu 5 point on the lung meridian becomes the sedation point and the Lu 11 point becomes the grandchild point.

Only the element point remains. Another name for the element point is the horary point. When using element points, you should use the needle with a tonifying or sedating maneuver. Element points attract or repel energy from the organ in the opposite direction according to the organ clock. If you want it to pull, you need to use it with a tonifying maneuver, if you want it to push, you need to use it with a sedating maneuver. One of the organs located in the opposite direction according to the organ clock is the Yang organ and the other is the Yin organ. For example, the organ in the exact opposite direction of the lung according to the organ clock is the bladder (Figure 65). If the Lu 8 point, which is the element point on the lung meridian, is tonified, the Yang energy in the bladder will change polarity and pass to the lungs as Yin energy. If sedated, the Yin energy in the lungs will change polarity and be pushed into the bladder as Yang energy. Therefore, if the element point in the Yin meridians is tonified, it only increases Yin; if it is sedated, it only decreases Yin. If the element point in the Yang meridians is tonified, it only increases Yang; if it is sedated, it only decreases Yang. There is no rule that the element point is only used in horary time. It can also be used at different times. Thambirajah says that the simultaneous use of element points with the horari clock is much more effective than acupuncture performed at other times. For example, tonification of the Lu 8 point to increase the Yin energy of the lungs, if done between 3 and 5 a.m., is many times more effective than when done at other times.

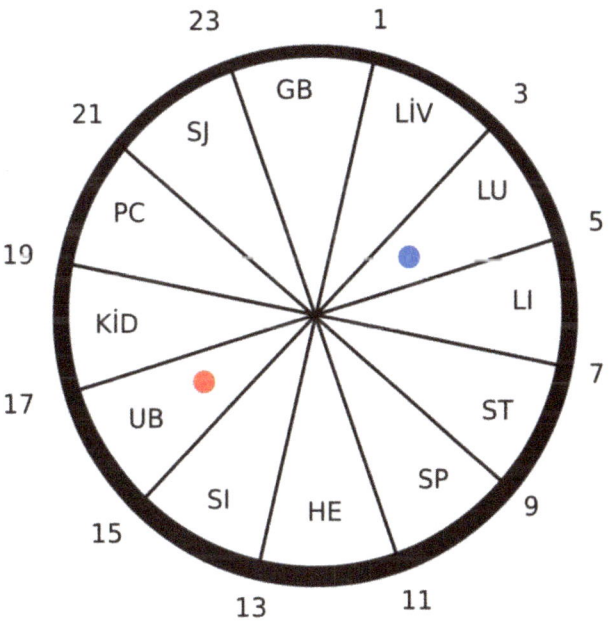

Figure 65: Organ clock

For friends who are just at the beginning of the science of acupuncture, it will not be easy to remember which organ is in the opposite direction according to the organ clock. Therefore, if you, the reader of this book, are in this situation, that is, if you are just learning this science, when using the element point, ignore the information from which organ the point draws energy. When you use this point on the Yin meridians, know that if you tone you increase the patient's Yin energy, if you calm it, you decrease it. When you use this point on the Yang meridians, if you tonify, you increase the patient's Yang energy, and if you sedate, you decrease it. This will be enough. It will be enough for a practitioner at the beginning of this path to know this for now. As you gain experience in this science, knowing the organs in the opposite direction according to the organ clock can enable you to kill two birds with one stone. For example, in a patient with Yang dominant chronic low back pain and a dry cough due to allergic rhinitis, tonifying the Lu 8 element point can relieve both complaints together. If the Lu 8 point is tonified, the Yang energy in the bladder will change polarity and pass to the lungs as Yin energy. The decrease in Yang in the bladder will cause relief in lower back pain, and the increased Yin energy in the lungs will cause a decrease in cough.

FIVE SHU POINTS OF THE LARGE INTESTINE MERIDIAN

The five Shu points on the Yang meridians are named from distal to proximal, not in the same order as on the Yin meridians. Let's draw an imaginary picture again to remember this order. Imagine a tree being watered by a metal armature. Let this tree be planted directly in the ground, not in a pot. Imagine that the sun's rays settling between the tree and the ground also catch your eye (Figure 66). In this case, the order of the five Shu points on the Yang meridians will be metal, water, wood, fire, earth.

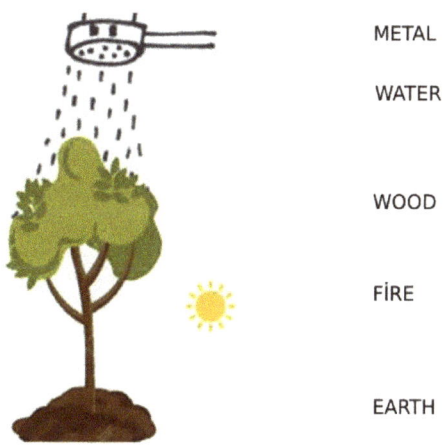

Figure 66: Naming order of the five shu points on the yang meridians

After this preliminary information, let's now write down the five shu points on the large intestine meridian in order. The large intestine meridian starts from the tip of the index finger on the hand and ends at the head. It starts with the number 1 because its starting point is at the tip of the finger.

The first three points were in order. We placed the points LI 1, LI, LI 3 in order. The fourth dot does not follow the order (LI 5), the fifth point does not follow the order (LI 11). In this case, LI 5 and LI 11 points are memorized. Now let's name the points. We were starting the yang meridians from metal. LI1 point becomes metal, LI 2 point becomes water, LI 3 point becomes wood, LI 5 point becomes fire, LI 11 point becomes earth point (Figure 67).

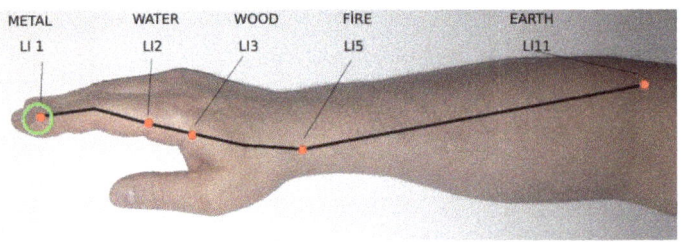

Figure 67: Five shu points of the large intestine meridian

The first thing we had to find was the element point. Since the large intestine belongs to the metal element, LI 1 point becomes the element point. The point before the element point was the mother point or tonification point. When you look at the meridian, you can say that there is no point before LI 1 point. If you think of the meridian as a circle, you will understand that the point before it is the LI 11 point. In this case, LI 11 point becomes the tonification point. The LI 5 point before the tonification point becomes the grandmother point. The point after the element point was the son point, and the point after that was the grandson point. We said that the son and grandson points are the points that close the tap. In this case, LI 2 point becomes the son point and LI 3 point becomes the grandson point.

Thus, we have completed the five shu points on the lung and large intestine meridians, which are the two organs of the metal element. Before moving on to examples of clinical use of these points, I would like to touch upon some points that I consider important for understanding the subject.

There are two ways to increase the Yin of the Yang organs. Before reading the rest of the sentence, I want you to look at the figure below and guess these two ways based on the figure (Figure 68). Either the grandmother point on the meridian of the Yang organ is used, or it is increased indirectly through its sister organ. As seen in the figure, sister organs are like communicating vessels. Through deep connections, the energy change in one of them passes to the sister organ in a short time. Considering this information, if I increase the Yin of the Yang organ's sister Yin organ, I will indirectly increase the Yin of the Yang organ, and this second way is the more frequently preferred way.

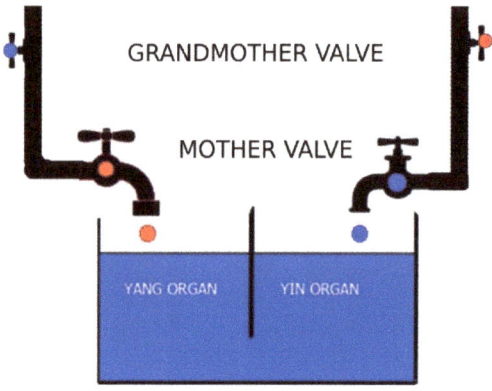

Figure 68: Representation of mother and grandmother points on meridians

Let's make the same sentence for Yin organs. There are two ways to increase the Yang of the Yin organs. Either the grandmother point on the meridian of the Yin organ is used, or the Yang of its sister organ is increased, thus indirectly increasing the Yang of the Yin organ.

In this system we will explain, there is only one way to reduce the Yin of the Yang organs and the Yang of the Yin organs. This process is done through the sister organ. For example, if you want to reduce the Yang of the lung, you must reduce the Yang of the large intestine, the sister organ of the lung. In other words, since the hot water fountain opening to the metal pool is the large intestine meridian, this process is done through the large intestine meridian. If you want to reduce the Yin of the large intestine, then you should turn off the cold water fountain that opens to the metal pool. So you have to close the lung meridian.

You will understand the subject much better after the example cases we will give now.

SAMPLE CASES ABOUT THE METAL ELEMENT

EXAMPLE CASE 1 (ACUTE SINUSITIS):

During the examination of the patient, who had complaints of cough, hoarseness, phlegm, and yellow-green nasal discharge for 2 days, we saw a partially yellowish, thick tongue fur and felt his pulse as a slippery pulse. What should our treatment plan be like for the patient?

With his symptoms, the patient says that the faulty pool is the lung pool. We have described phlegm cases as excess dampness and the body's increase in Yang against this dampness. The thickening and partial yellowing of the tongue fur also indicates this. The fact that the complaint has been around for 2 days and the tongue-pulse findings indicate that the case is excess. This means that both the hot water fountain and the cold water fountain of the pool are flowing excessively. In this case, it is necessary to turn off the cold water and hot water fountains together. So we need to sedate both the Yin and Yang of the lung.

I can use the son or grandson points (Lu 5 and Lu 11) over the lung meridian to turn off the cold water fountain. I use the large intestine meridian to reduce the Yang of the lung. So I turn off the hot water fountain going to the metal pool. For this purpose, I use the son and grandson points (Li 2, Li 3) on the large intestine meridian. Thus, I reduce the Yang of the large intestine and indirectly the Yang of the lungs. In such cases of phlegm, it would be appropriate to use points on the spleen and stomach organs, which are responsible for the transport and transformation of fluids. Although this is out of our scope for now, it would be appropriate to add Sp 9 and St 44 points to remove dampness and heat.

EXAMPLE CASE 2 (FREQUENTLY RECURRENT UPPER RESPIRATORY TRACT INFECTION):

The patient, who describes frequent sweating and recurrent upper respiratory tract infections, rapid fatigue, and frequent hoarseness and cough, says that his complaints intensify between 3 and 5 in the afternoon. On examination, the tongue fur was normal and the tongue body was swollen. His pulse was thin and weak, like cotton thread, on the right side in the distal position. What should our treatment plan be like for the patient?

The patient's symptoms and findings indicate that the faulty pool is the lung. Pulse and tongue findings indicate lung Qi deficiency. In lung Qi deficiency, spontaneous sweating is observed day and night, as in lung Yang deficiency. Since Wei Qi is weak in these patients, sweat pores remain open and spontaneous sweats and a history of frequent infections occur. Every organ has hours when its energy is at its maximum. Lung energy is maximum between 3-5 pm at night and minimum between 3-5 pm in the afternoon (Figure 69). That's why the complaints of patients with Lung Qi deficiency increase between 3-5 pm.

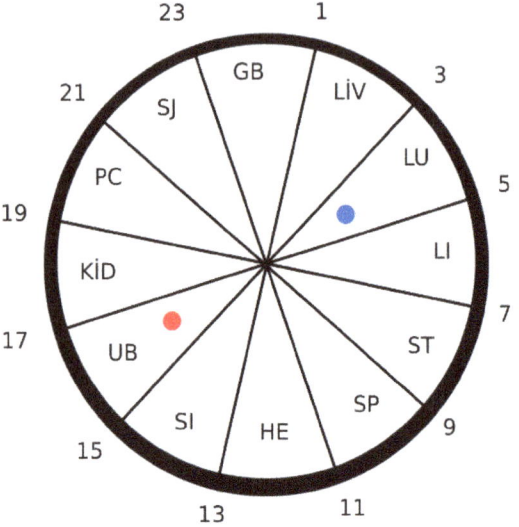

Figure 69: Organ clock

In this patient, lung Yin and Yang should be increased in a balanced manner. In other words, 1 or 2 cold water fountains and 1 or 2 hot water fountains should be opened. The tonification point (Lu 9) can be used to increase Lung Yin. If you want to open a second cold water fountain, the element point (Lu 8) is used with the tonifying maneuver. We can increase lung Yang in two ways. It can be increased either indirectly by using the grandmother point (Lu 10) on the lung meridian, or, more commonly, through the large intestine meridian. For this purpose, the tonification point of the large intestine (LI 11) can be used. In some reference books, the LI 11 point is called the immunomodulatory point. Even though I do not like such naming, I am quoting it in the hope that it may help understand the truth. So, since the LI 11 point increases the Yang of the large intestine and indirectly the lungs, this feature of the point was tried to be emphasized with this description.

In the first chapters of the book, we said that the criticisms of the five shu points would be touched upon when appropriate. The fact that the LI 11 point is used in practice to reduce fever is one of the most important criticisms of these points. Although LI 11 point is the tonification point, it is said that it has an antipyretic effect. We explain this as follows. Yin and Yang are in constant transformation in the universe. After the night reaches perfection, it emerges during the day. After the winter season ends, the summer season emerges. We have previously said that among the Yang meridians, the meridian with the highest Yang energy is the large intestine meridian. In febrile illness, Yang energy moves towards peak point in the meridian where Yang is highest. By using the LI 11 point, it is easier for Yang to reach the peak point, thus the process of Yang turning into Yin is accelerated. Therefore, in patients where the LI 11 point is used, the fever first increases and then decreases. It is not recommended to use the dot on children and the elderly for this purpose. Likewise, its use is not recommended in cases where the fever is prolonged and dryness symptoms occur due to fluid loss due to sweating.

EXAMPLE CASE 3 (ASTHMA AND CHRONIC CONSTIPATION)

The patient had complaints of cough, shortness of breath, and hoarseness for years, and these complaints increased in dry weather. His symptoms were relieved, especially when he went on vacation to coastal residential areas. He also describes additional symptoms such as nasal dryness, occasional nosebleeds, and constipation. He says he sweats a lot, especially at night. On examination, we felt the right anterior pulse as weak and superficial. The tongue fur is missing in places, the remaining parts are yellowed, the tongue body looks dry. What should our treatment plan be like for the patient?

The patient's symptoms and findings indicate that the faulty pool is the lung. Pulse and tongue findings indicate lung Yin deficiency. The pool is warm, but empty. In cases where the lung pool is hot, constipation is frequently observed as the large intestine pool will also be hot. As we said before, night sweats are observed in the presence of Yin deficiency in any organ, not just the lungs. All we need to do for this patient is to turn on the cold water fountain. For this purpose, it will be sufficient to use the element point of the lung (Lu 8) with a tonifying maneuver and the tonification point (Lu 9). These are points that balance energy and perform root treatment. We can use local point. For example, we can use St 25 and Sp 15 points as local points for constipation. We can add Lu1 and UB 13 points for the lungs, and LI 20 and Yintang points for nasal dryness as local points. Even if we never use these local points, the patient's complaints will usually be relieved. Of course, we never talked about acupuncture session intervals. As far as I can see in the reference books I have read, acupuncture sessions are applied every day in China for both chronic insufficiency and acute excess cases. I do chronic insufficiency cases 2 sessions a week, 10 in total. I do it every day in cases of chronic insufficiency with recurrent attacks and if the attacks are very severe. I also treat acute excess cases every day. I end the sedation process of the patients I sedated as soon as their symptoms are relieved. Because long-term sedation causes organ functions to slow down. For example, if you sedate the large intestine for a long time, the patient may come to you with frequent recurrences of infection.

EXAMPLE CASE 4 (ULCERATIVE COLITIS AND ASTHMA):

The patient, diagnosed with ulcerative colitis, came to us with complaints of abdominal pain and bloody and mucusy stools for 2 days. He says that this complaint occurs occasionally in attacks, and that he defecates like goat poop between attacks. During the examination, it was observed that the tongue fur was missing in places and the remaining part was yellowing, the tongue body was thin and dry, and there were cracks in the anterior part. During pulse examination, a superficial, thin, guitar string-like pulse was detected in the right anterior position. What should our treatment plan be like for the patient?

Our target pool is the large intestine. There are hot pool findings. Chronic case but in the recurrent attack phase. In chronic cases that progress with attacks, we expect the Yin Yang diagram during the attack as one increased and the other decreased. The tongue finding indicates yin deficiency. The pulse finding also indicates that Yin cannot control Yang, therefore there is Yang hyperactivity that develops on the basis of Yin deficiency. We expect the Yin Yang diagram in this patient to be just like the Yin Yang diagram we drew in chronic recurrent gastritis (Figure 70).

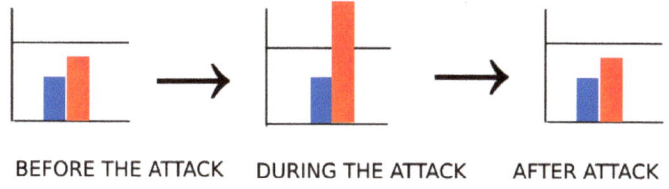

BEFORE THE ATTACK   DURING THE ATTACK   AFTER ATTACK

Figure 70: Yin Yang diagram before, during and after an ulcerative colitis attack

A cold water fountain should be turned on in this patient we saw during an attack. If the patient's complaint is relieved, there is no need to do anything additional. If it does not provide relief, the hot water fountain should be turned off. To turn on the cold water fountain, it is sufficient to use the element point of the lung (Lu 8) with a tonifying maneuver and the tonification point (Lu 9). The son point (LI 2), or the grandson point (LI 3) of the large intestine meridian can be used to turn off the hot water fountain. The treatment of the patient after the attack will be to open two cold water fountains and one hot water fountain. In other words, the tonification point of the large intestine (LI 11) can be added to Lu 9 and Lu 8 points.

Our treatment method will be no different from this for an asthma patient who comes to you with a clinical appearance that is restless and cyanotic, wheezing so that the respiratory sounds can be heard from outside, accompanied by strong coughs, and whose tongue and pulse examination is just like this ulcerative colitis patient.

There are two types of asthma. First, this is the type of asthma where the pool is hot. These attacks are severe. During the attack, bronchoconstriction is severe, and a whistle-like sound may be heard during breathing, which can be heard even from outside. The patient looks extremely restless and the cough is dry. Night sweats occur due to yin deficiency. The other is damp-cold type asthma, where the pool is cold. They do not have such severe attacks. There are periods when the patient just gets better and worse. Cough increases in humid weather, breathing sounds cannot be heard from outside, wheezing, rales and crepitations are recorded with a stethoscope. In the type of asthma where the pool is dry, the patient's breathing sounds are completely normal between attacks, but in humidity type asthma, wheezing, rales and crepitations can be detected with a stethoscope between attacks. Although it is not correct to define a period as an attack period, there are only periods when the patient is better and worse. In humidity-type asthma, one or two hot water fountains that heat the pool and points on the spleen-stomach meridian are preferred for the transport of liquids.

I would like to draw the reader's attention to one point. While TCM can use different points in a disease that Western Medicine calls asthma, it can use the same point in two diseases it calls different names.

EXAMPLE CASE 5 (SHOULDER PAIN):

The patient has been complaining of pain in the front of the shoulder on the left side for 2 years. This pain occurs when he moves his shoulder. The patient, who does not have much pain at night, cannot clearly say whether his pain increases or decreases by applying hot or cold. On examination, it is observed that active and passive joint range of motion has decreased. It was observed that there was a partial loss of the tongue fur, the color of the remaining part was white, the tongue body appeared pale and dry, and there were cracks in places. His pulse was observed to be weak and superficial in the right anterior and middle positions. What should our treatment plan be like for the patient?

The patient shows his pain by describing the area rather than the meridian course. We will use the meridians in the anterior of the extremities in the treatment, as they show the anterior area of the shoulder (Figure 71). Symptoms and findings such as pain occurring with movement, loss of tongue fur, cracked and dry appearance in the tongue body, and shallow pulse indicate that the pool is hot.

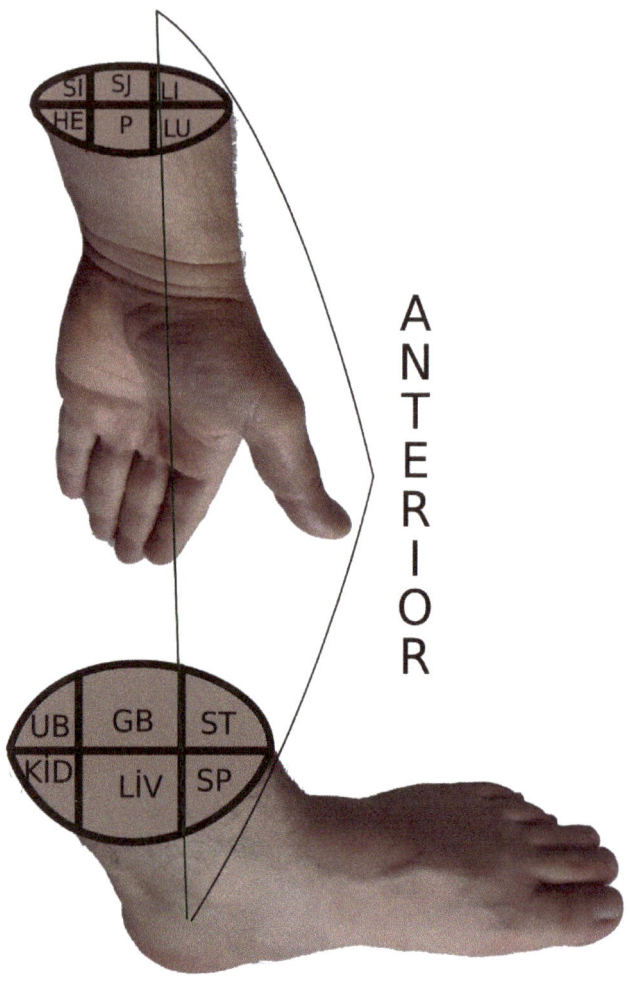

Figure 71: Meridians in the anterior extremities

The duration of the complaint, symptoms and signs indicate that it is a case of deficiency, that is, empty heat. The whiteness of the patient's remaining tongue fur and the paleness of the tongue body give clues that Yang is also lower than normal (Figure 72).

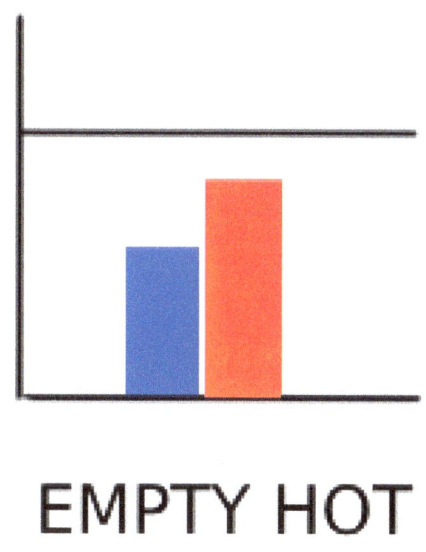

EMPTY HOT

Figure 72: Empty heat where Yang also falls

In the treatment of the patient, opening one hot water tap and two cold water taps will be sufficient. The tonification point of the large intestine meridian (LI 11) can be used as a hot water tap, the element point of the lung meridian (Lu 8) can be used with a tonifying maneuver and the tonification point (Lu 9) can be used as a cold water tap. It would be good if the same procedure is done for the stomach and spleen meridians in the lower extremities. Although we have not yet explained the meridians of the earth element, let's briefly mention them. The element point (St 36) on the stomach meridian is suitable for turning on the hot water fountain, but let us also say that the St 38 point, which is not among the five element points in practice, is more recommended than the St 36 point for shoulder pain. The tonification point (Sp 2) and the element point (Sp 3) are also suitable points for the cold water fountain, which we recommend to have two.

EXAMPLE CASE 6 (LATERAL EPICONDYLITIS):

The patient, who has been experiencing pain in his left elbow for 15-20 days when opening and closing a door handle or carrying a load, states that his pain is relieved when he applies ice. On examination, the area between the lateral epicondyle and the lateral end of the cubital fold is detected as painful and tender by palpation. No abnormalities are detected in the tongue and pulse examination. What should our treatment plan be like for the patient?

It appears that the patient's faulty pool is the large intestine. In acute diseases related to the meridian course, there may be no specific findings on tongue and pulse examination. The fact that the patient's pain occurs with movement, is relieved by applying ice, the pool is warm, and the history is shorter than 1 month also indicates that it is excess.

The only thing to do in this patient is to turn off the hot water fountain. For this purpose, it would be appropriate to use the son (LI 2) and grandson (LI 3) points on the large intestine meridian. A question like "Can we use LI 11 as a local point?" may come to mind. Since the LI 11 point is a tonification point, if it is needled and left, it increases Yang even more. If it is to be used, it should be used with a sedating maneuver.

Since tendons are tissue related to the wood element, it would be good to include the grandson point (Gb 34) on the gallbladder meridian in the treatment. "Why was the grandson point suggested and not the son point", we would say that the Gb 34 point is not only the grandson point on the gallbladder meridian, but also one of the eight influence points. This is the influential point of the tendons.

Examples of the clinical use of the five shu points on the lung and large intestine meridians can be increased further, but I believe this will be enough to understand the subject. Now let's examine the five shu points of the earth element.

STOMACH MERIDIAN FIVE SHU POINTS

The stomach meridian starts from the head and ends at the lateral corner of the second toe. The point where it ends at the foot is St 45. The first three points go in order: St 45, St 44, St 43. The fourth and fifth points go by skipping, the fourth point is St 41 at the ankle, the fifth point is St 36 around the knee. Now let's do the naming. Yang meridians started with metal. St 45 is called metal, St 44 is called water, St 43 is called wood, St 41 is fire, St 36 is called earth. The first point we would find was the element point. In this case, St 36 point is the element point. The one before the element point is the tonification point (St 41), and the one before it is the grandmother point (St 43). The point after the element point is the son point (St 45), and the point after that "St 44" is the grandson point (Figure 73).

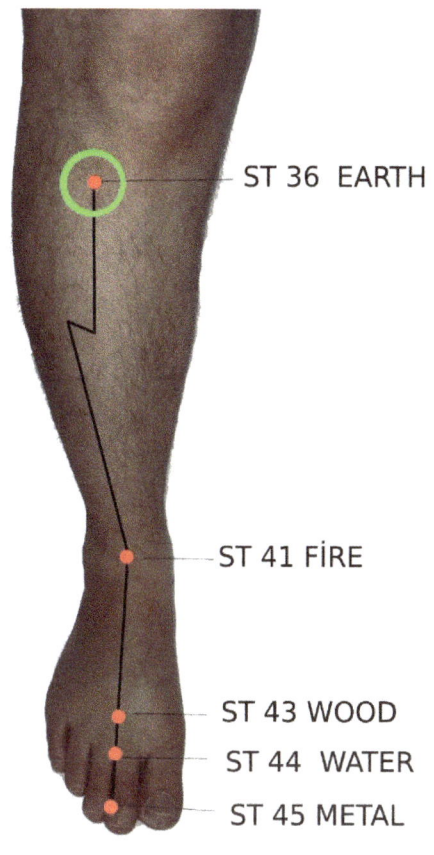

Figure 73: Stomach meridian five shu points

St 36 point is the element point of the meridian. This point is used very frequently in practical applications. If a single point is to be used in cases where the stomach will be tonified, the St 36 point is generally preferred rather than the tonification point. Thambirajah does not recommend using this point with a sedating maneuver, but Giovanni says it can. It is the most important of the points that increase general energy. It is the empiric distal point used for the abdominal region.

FIVE SHU POINTS OF THE SPLEEN MERIDIAN

The spleen meridian starts from the medial corner of the big toe and ends in the thorax. Since the starting point is the fingertip, it starts with the number 1. The first three points go in order: Sp 1, Sp 2, Sp 3. The fourth and fifth points go by skipping, the fourth point is "Sp 5" around the ankle, the fifth point is "Sp 9" around the knee. The first point we had to find was the element point. Spleen Since , it belongs to the earth element, the Sp 3 point becomes the element point, the "Sp 2 point" before it is the tonification point, and the Sp 5 point after the Element point is the son point. Sp 9 is the grandchild point (Figure 74)

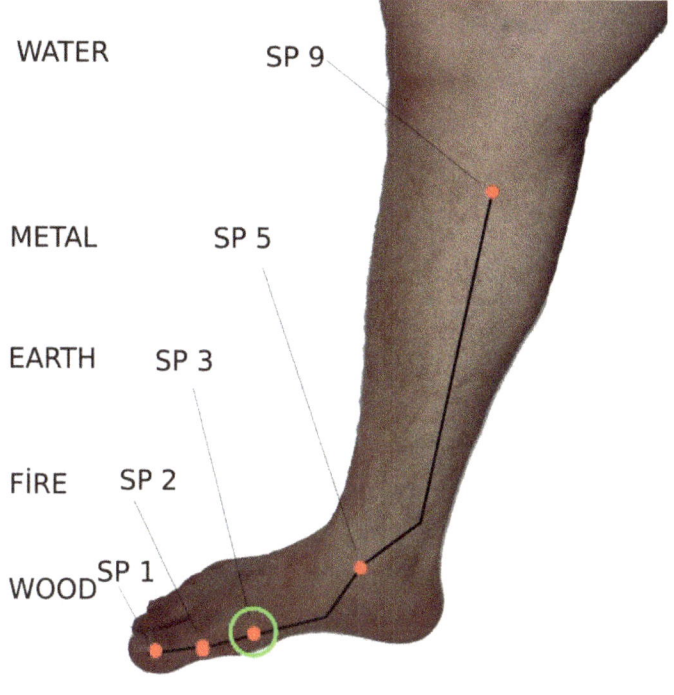

Figure 74: Spleen meridian five shu points

The son point and grandson points are the points that turn off the tap. The sedation point "Sp 5", being a metal point, sends Yin energy to the metal element, and the grandson point "Sp 9", being a water point, sends Yin energy to the water element, thus turning off the tap. Sp 9 point is called the "Lasix point" because it sends Yin energy to the kidney. This nomenclature can sometimes lead to misapplications in the clinic, such as using the Sp 9 point in every case of edema. In cases of edema secondary to stomach and splenic deficiency, should we perform tonification or sedation? I have already mentioned this issue in the tongue examination, but let's repeat it because it is relevant. Tonification is performed in cases of deficiency and sedation in cases of excess. Dampness or phlegm secondary to stomach-spleen deficiency is an excessive condition, but since it develops on the basis of deficiency, the pulse is checked. If the pulse is weak, tonification is performed, if it is strong, sedation is performed. Here, in cases of edema secondary to spleen-stomach deficiency, if the pulse is strong, Sp 9 point can be used, if it is weak, it is not correct to use Sp 9 point. In such cases, tonifying points are selected over the stomach and spleen, the fluid transfer function of the spleen is activated and the recovery of edema is left to time. With this type of treatment, the recovery of the edema will be later than in cases of pure excessive edema where the Sp 9 point is used in the treatment. However, in cases where there is a combination of deficiency and excess and the pulse is weak, the use of the Sp 9 point will not improve the clinic.

Since the spleen meridian is a Yin meridian, the Sp 1 grandmother point on it increases the Yang of the organ. If moxa is applied to the point, this effect is greater.

SAMPLE CASES RELATED TO EARTH ELEMENT

EXAMPLE CASE 1 (CHRONIC GASTRITIS):

On examination of the patient who had epigastric burning for years, especially after heavy meals, the tongue corpus was swollen and tooth marks were present, anteriorly there was hyperemia in the papillae, and the tongue fur was partially thick and yellowed (Figure 75). The pulse was weak, superficial and slightly thick in the right middle position. What should be our treatment plan in this patient?

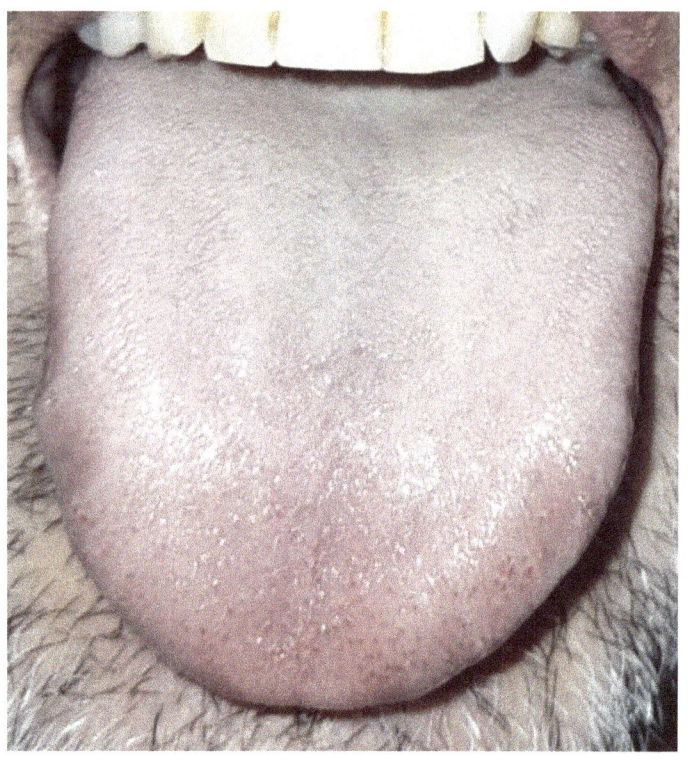

Figure 75: Tongue image

Our first case example of the earth element is a difficult one. Epigastric pain indicates that the faulty pool is the stomach pool. A weak and superficial pulse is a sign that the pool is empty and hot. However, a thick pulse, no loss of tongue fur, on the contrary, thickening and yellowing, and a swollen appearance of the tongue body indicate phlegm that develops secondary to deciency. As we have just said, in cases where excess and deficiency occur together and the pulse is weak, tonification should be performed. In this case where the pool is hot, it would be appropriate to open two cold water fountains and one hot water fountain. For this purpose, although the combination of Sp 2, Sp 3 and St 36 points generally relieves the symptoms of burning in the stomach and epigastric pain in a short time, it will take a long time for the phlegm to improve. Although the hyperemic papilla in the anterior part of the tongue corpus indicates that the metal pool is hot, it is beneficial to add the element point (Lu 8) or tonification point (Lu 9) of the lung meridian to the treatment, even if the patient does not have any symptoms of the metal pool such as cough or constipation. Although such patients do not have any complaints about the large intestine or lungs, there may be symptoms that the patient does not care about, such as dryness of the skin and nose, and dandruff at the roots of the hair.

EXAMPLE CASE 2 (LYMPHEDEMA):

The patient, who had mastectomy surgery due to breast cancer approximately 10 years ago, developed lymphedema in her right arm 3 months ago. In the tongue examination, the tongue corpus appeared swollen with tooth marks, and no other noticeable change was detected except for a wide cleft in the middle extending from the central to the anterior, called the "Heart cleft" (Figure 76). During pulse examination, the middle pulse on the right side was felt as weak, superficial and thick. What should our treatment plan be like for the patient?

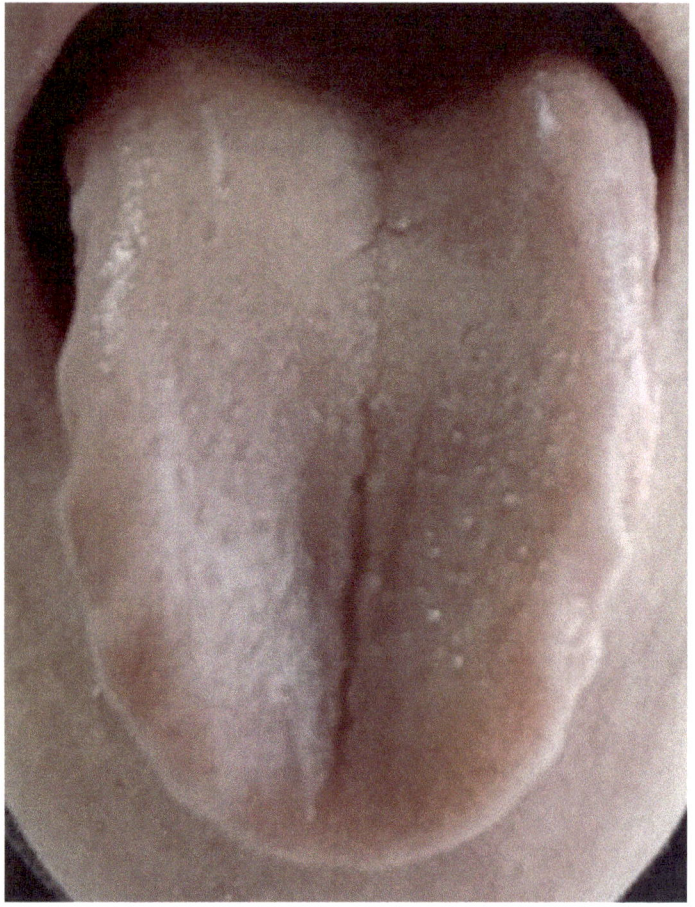

Figure 76: Tongue image

There are two reasons why I included this patient among the earth element sample cases. The first is the location of the breast tissue on the course of the stomach meridian, and the second is the presence of edema in the upper extremity. The presence of edema in the body makes the earth element a target pool. The presence of a "Heart Cleft" in the patient's tongue body is a sign of stomach and heart Yin deficiency. The presence of tooth marks and edematous appearance in the tongue body indicate dampness accumulation secondary to spleen yin deficiency. A shallow and weak pulse indicates empty heat, while a thick pulse is evidence of the presence of dampness. In this patient, just like in the previous patient, two cold water fountains (Sp 2, Sp 3) and one hot water fountain (St 36) are appropriate. For heart Yin deficiency, it would be good to open one or two cold water fountains over the heart meridian.

EXAMPLE CASE 3 (REPEAT ANKLE SPRAIN):

The patient described a recurrent inward sprain of the right ankle, which resulted in prolonged loss of work. No significant findings were found except for a swollen and moist appearance of the tongue corpus and the presence of teeth marks. His pulse was felt as deep and weak. The thickness of the pulse was perceived as normal. What should our treatment plan be like for the patient?

The patient did not describe a specific meridian and the tone of the medial side muscles of the right ankle was felt to be decreased compared to the left. It is not easy to identify the defective pool in this patient. Because of the association of the muscle tissue with the earth element and the supporting tongue and pulse findings, we decided that the defective pool was an earth pool. Unfortunately, if this first step is wrong, we will not be able to help the patient. The deep pulse and tongue findings suggested that the pool was cold, while the weak pulse and the prolonged duration of the complaint suggested a case of insufficiency. We opened 2 hot water fountains in this patient. We needled the St 36 point and applied moxa to the Sp 1 point. After 10 sessions of application, the patient never had a sprain again (patient with follow-up that we have been communicating for 5-6 years).

EXAMPLE CASE 4 (ACUTE TONSILLITIS):

During the examination of the patient, who had been complaining of severe sore throat, painful swelling under the chin, fever and intense sweating for two days, hyperemia and exudate in the tonsils and submandibular tender lymphadenopathy were observed. From a Western medical perspective, we diagnosed the patient with cryptic tonsillitis. The patient's tongue fur appeared thickened and yellowed, and the tongue corpus appeared slightly hyperemic in the anterior aspect (Figure 77). The pulse was felt as a slippery pulse in the anterior and middle positions on the right side. What should our treatment plan be for the patient?

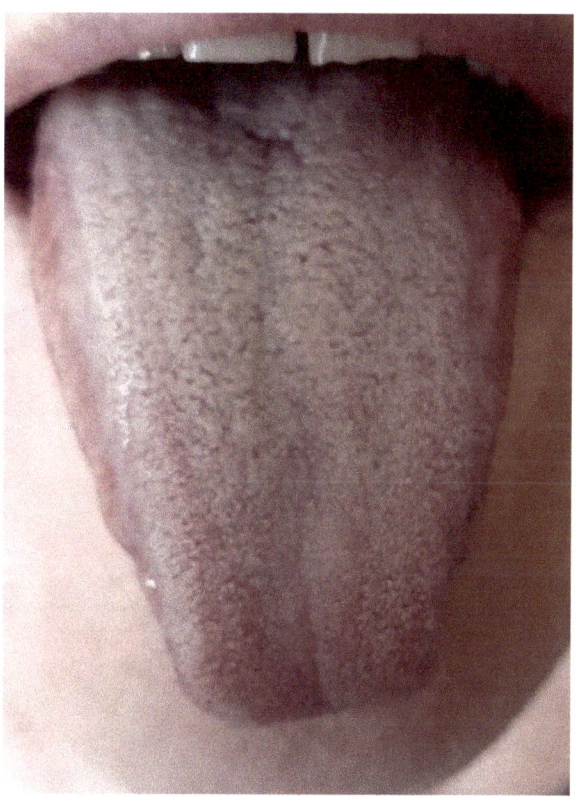

Figure 77: Tongue image

Before evaluating the case, I think it would be right to give a brief explanation about external pathogens. According to the TCM, there are six external pathogens: "Wind, cold, heat, dampness, dryness and summer heat". Among these six pathogens, wind acts as a mediator for other pathogens to enter the body. Cold and dampness can be grouped under the umbrella of Yin pathogens, and heat and dryness under the umbrella of Yang pathogens. Imagine that in the heat of summer, when people are exposed to the sun in damp clothes, dampness pathogen and heat pathogen cause disease together.

As we have said before, since the anterior side of the body has Yang ming meridians, where Yang energy is most concentrated, the cold pathogen enters the body from the back and causes symptoms such as neck and back pain in the posterior region of the body in the early period. The hot pathogen, on the other hand, enters the body from the anterior side and causes symptoms such as tonsillitis, lymphadenitis and sinusitis in the anterior region of the body in the early stages. However, do not be misunderstood, if both pathogens cannot be removed from the body, symptoms related to the meridians in the anterior, posterior or lateral parts of the body may occur in the later stages of the disease. There is also an early stage in which the pathogen lodges between the skin and muscles, which is called the external stage. Since Wei Qi, which protects the body against external pathogens, is located between the skin and muscles, and since Wei Qi is under the control of the lung, whether the pathogen is a Yin pathogen or a Yang pathogen, symptoms related to the lung such as cough, hoarseness, and runny nose can be observed in the early stage of the disease. In the external stage of Yang pathogen, there may be no tongue findings. There may be hyperemia only in the anterior tongue corpus. But usually Yang pathogen progresses very rapidly. If the body responds to the Yang pathogen by increasing its humidity, thickening and yellowing of the tongue rust will soon appear. If the Yin pathogen is in the external stage, white thick tongue fur forms. If the disease progresses and the body responds by increasing its temperature, the white and thick tongue fur starts to turn yellow.

Again, before introducing the topic, I think it would be useful to explain the difference between what is referred to as "Damp-heat" in the reference books and phlegm. In phlegm, the body responds to the dampness pathogen by increasing body temperature, whereas in "Damp-heat", the body responds to the heat pathogen by increasing body dampness (Figure 78). As a result, in both cases, heat and dampness excesses are combined. In both, the tongue fur is thick and yellow. In both cases the pulse is slippery.

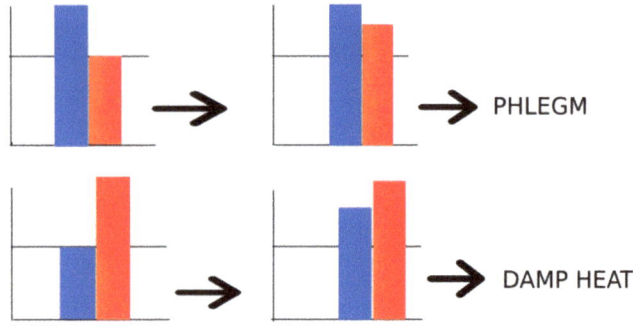

Figure 78: Difference between phlegm and damp heat

In the treatment of both phlegm and "damp heat", hot and cold water taps are turned off together. A second opinion is that since the primary factor in phlegm is moisture, and heat is only a reactionary reaction to it, only the moisture is removed. The opposite is the case with damp heat. Here, the primary factor is heat, and only heat is removed because the damp reacts against it, according to this second opinion, which says that if the primary factor is removed, the reactionary response automatically disappears.

In the examination of the tongue in such acute infectious conditions, attention should be focused on the tongue fur in order to obtain information about the nature of the external pathogen. Yellowing of the tongue fur indicates that the pool is hot and thickening indicates excessive dampness. The pulse also supports this. I interpret such cases as cases of "Damp heat" due to Yang pathogen invasion into the Yang ming channels in the anterior part of the body. Therefore, I propose to close at least one of the hot and cold water fountains that open into the pools anterior to the extremities. For this purpose, the son or grandson points of the large intestine (LI 2, LI 3), the son or grandson points of the stomach (St 45, St 44) are the points where we can close the hot water fountain. The son and grandson points of the lung (Lu 5, Lu 11), the son and grandson points of the spleen (Sp 5, Sp 9) are also points where we can turn off the cold water fountain.

Assuming that the case studies of the earth element are sufficient for understanding the subject, we will move on to the organs of the fire element. There are four organs in the fire element. The heart, small intestine, pericardium and sanjiao. Let's first see their five shu points and then move on to the case studies.

HEART MERIDIAN FIVE SHU POINTS

The cardiac meridian starts from the axilla and ends at the radial corner of the little finger. Its termination point is the He 9 point. The first three points go in order: He 9, He 8, He 7. The fourth and fifth points go by skipping, the fourth point is He 4 around the wrist, the fifth point is He 3 around the elbow. The first point we had to find was the element point. Since the heart belongs to the fire element, the He 8 point becomes the element point. The one before it is the "He 9 point" tonification point, and the one before that is the "He 3 point" grandmother point. The next He 7 point after the element point is the son point, and the next He 4 point after that is the grandson point (Figure 79).

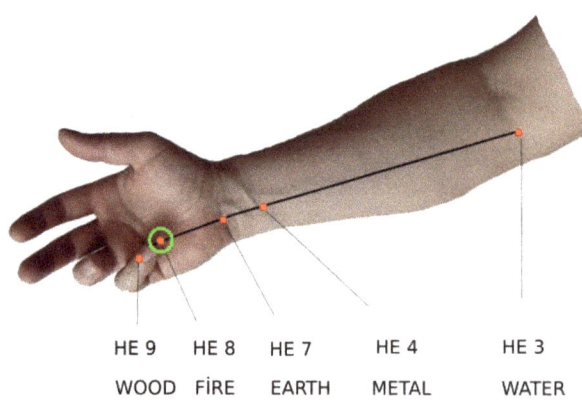

Figure 79: Five shu points on the heart meridian

One of the criticisms of the five shu points by some Western writers is directed at the He 9 and P 9 points, which we will discuss in a moment. The criticism is that although He 9 and P 9 points are tonification points, they are used in the clinic for sedation in diseases such as fever reduction, hypertensive attack and cardiovascular collapse. Again, some Western authors say that the first two shu points are used for sedation even though they are tonification points. As far as I can see, the reason these authors think this way is that they think there is no other way to lower fever and blood pressure other than sedation. Tonifying the opposite of something is also a form of sedation. So the opposite of heat is cold. By tonifying cold, you sedate the heat. So both the He 9 point and the P 9 point are points that open the faucet on the Yin meridian, so they cool the pool. Turning down the hot water tap is not the only way to cool the pool. In cardiovascular collapse, it is necessary to tonify organ function. I think the criticism here is that because of the acute nature of the event, the procedure is perceived as a sedation procedure. The way to revive a dysfunctional heart is, of course, to tonify the Yin and Yang of the organ together.

We said that the He 8 point is the element point of the meridian. This is a useful point in the acute attack period of migraine patients. The fire element is the son of the wood element. In migraine patients, the fire pool is usually hot. According to the organ clock, the gallbladder is located in the opposite direction of the heart (Figure 80). So when we tonify the He 8 point, the Yang of the gallbladder changes polarity and flows into the heart as Yin energy. Therefore, the Yin of the heart is increased and the Yang of the gallbladder is decreased.

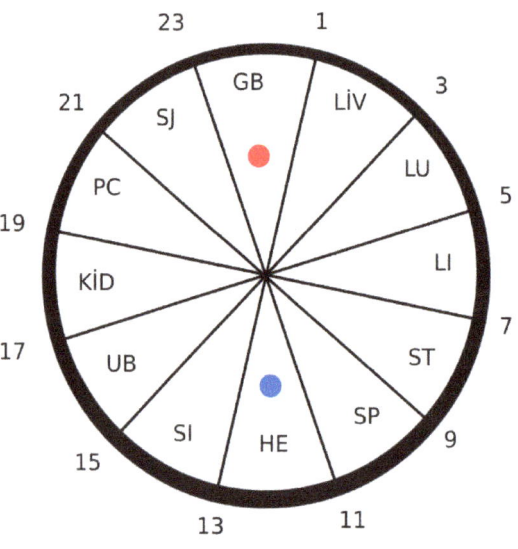

Figure 80: Organ clock

He 7 and He 4 are the points that turn down the tap. In the yin meridians, the third point from the distal is the yuan point. Therefore, the He 7 point is both a yuan point and a sedation point. Therefore, because it is a Yuan point, it has the possibility of tonifying Yin energy and because it is a sedation point, it has the possibility of sedating Yin energy. Therefore, we need to manifest the desired effect through needle manipulation. In other words, if we want to tonify Yin energy, we need to use the needle with a tonifying maneuver, and if we want to sedate it, we need to use it with a sedating maneuver. The Chinese name for this point is Shenmen point. It means the gate of Shen. Giovanni makes the interesting point that this point can be used in mental retardation in children.

The He 3 point is the grandmother point. The grandmother point on the Yin meridian increases Yang. This point is also called the laughing point. This information may surprise the reader. Because I witness that the Yin of the heart is usually increased in the treatment of depression in our country. Depression can occur when both the Yang and Yin of the heart are deficient. Therefore, if the Yang of the heart is deficient, it is necessary to increase the Yang, and if the Yin of the heart is deficient, it is necessary to increase the Yin.

FIVE SHU POINTS OF THE SMALL INTESTINE MERIDIAN

The small intestine meridian starts at the ulnar nail corner of the little finger and ends at the head.

Because it starts at the fingertip, the five shu points start with the number 1. The first three points go in order: SI 1, SI 2, SI 3. The fourth and fifth point go by skipping. The fourth point is "SI 5" around the wrist and the fifth point is "SI 8" around the elbow. In the Yang meridians we were starting the first point with the metal. The first point we had to find was the element point. Since the small intestine belongs to the fire element, the SI 5 point becomes the element point. The one before it is the "SI 3 point" tonification point, and the one before that is the "SI 2 point" grandmother point. The next "SI 8 point" after the element point is the son point, and the next "SI 1 point" after that is the grandson point (Figure 81).

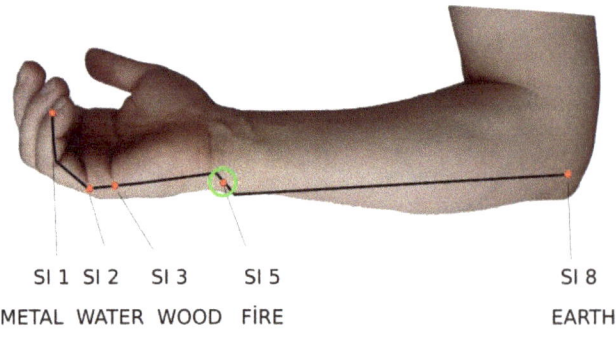

Figure 81: Five shu points on the small intestine meridian

SI 3 is the point that opens the hot water tap. It is also the confluent point of the Du meridian, one of the so-called extraordinary meridians. If we are using the SI 3 point not to increase the Yang of the small intestine meridian but to open the Du meridian, we need to use an additional point to help the body understand our intention. The use of this additional point varies from practitioner to practitioner, but since we plan to explain the five elements acupuncture in our book, we will not give detailed information on this subject.

SI 1 point is the grandchild point, that is, the point that closes the hot water tap. Giovanni states that this point is also used to increase breast milk after birth. The best way to increase breast milk is to do this with the points we choose through the earth element, since the breast tissue is located on the course of the stomach meridian and the stomach is the source of the postnatal Essence obtained through food. I can only comment on how the SI 1 point increases milk release. The emotional burden on the mother after birth may have warmed the heart pool. We have said before that all emotions ultimately affect the heart. Warming of the heart pool means warming of the blood. Blood, like milk, is a body fluid and body fluids can transform into each other. According to TCM, breast milk consists of blood. The heated heart pool also warms and dries the blood circulating in it. Therefore, milk formation decreases.

PERICHARD MERIDIAN FIVE SHU POINTS

The pericardial meridian starts from the thorax and ends at the tip of the middle finger. The point where it ends is point P9. The first three points go in order: P 9, P 8, P 7. The fourth and fifth points go by skipping, the fourth point is "P 5" around the wrist, the fifth point is "P 3" around the elbow. The first point we had to find was the element point. Pericardium Since it belongs to the fire element, the P 8 point becomes the element point, the "P 9 point" before it is the tonification point, and the P 7 point after the element point is the sedation point. P 5 point is the grandchild point (Figure 82).

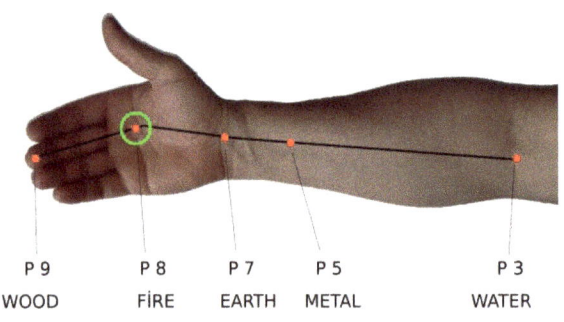

| P 9 | P 8 | P 7 | P 5 | P 3 |
| WOOD | FİRE | EARTH | METAL | WATER |

Figure 82: Five shu points of the pericardial meridian

P 9 point, like He 9 point, is the tonification point of the meridian. This point is a point that can be used safely in the treatment of hypertension in pregnant women. What we said for point He 9 is also valid for point P 9. P 9 and He 9 are mentioned among the useful points in cases where you want to cool the blood. Imagine the heat released by an organ contracting 72 times per minute. This heat is cooled by the blood passing through the heart. Therefore, when you want to cool the blood, points that cool the heart are used. This point is generally used by bleeding.

P8 point is the element point of the meridian. If it is tonified, you will only increase Yin; if it is sedated, you will only decrease Yin. The reader may not understand what I mean when we say "only increasing or decreasing Yin". For the tonification point in the Yin meridians, we said that it largely increases Yin and partly increases Yang. For element points, it is not possible to talk about such a thing. When I say it only increases Yin, I mean pure Yin increase. I mean it does not cause an increase in Yang. When I say it only reduces Yin, I mean pure Yin reduction. I mean, it does not cause a decrease in Yang. When the point is tonified, it draws Yang energy from the stomach in the opposite direction according to the organ clock, Yang energy changes polarity and turns into Yin energy and passes to the pericardium (Figure 83). These element points are very useful when both organ pools located in opposite directions are hot or when both organ pools are cold. For example, let's assume that a patient who has sleep disturbance, anxiety, tachycardia and hypertension due to the hot heart pool also has epigastric pain or frontal headache due to the hot stomach pool. If the P 8 point is tonified in this patient, the stomach pool will be cooled as it will draw the Yang energy in the stomach. At the same time, as Yang energy changes polarity and passes to the pericardium as Yin energy, the pericardium (and therefore the heart) is cooled.

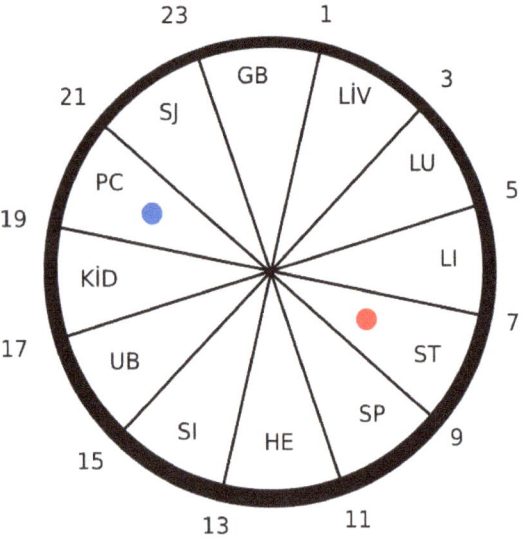

Figure 83: Stomach and pericardium according to the organ clock

Points P 7 and P 5 are the points that close the tap. The P 7 point, just like the He 7 point, is both a yuan point and a sedation point. P 5 point is the intersection point of the three Yin meridians on the arm. For this reason, both points have the possibility of tonifying Yin energy and sedating it. We need to make clear the effect we want with needle manipulation. In other words, if we want to tonify Yin energy, we need to use the needle with a tonifying maneuver, and if we want to sedate it, we need to use the needle with a sedating maneuver. Giovanni conveys an obscure information that the P 5 point is used as an empirical point in malaria. It is difficult to understand whether by malaria he means malaria or all febrile diseases. Since it is the intersection point of three Yin meridians, it seems more reasonable to refer to all febril diseases, as its tonification will strongly nourish Yin. Since P3 point is the grandmother point, it is the point that increases Yang on the Yin meridian.

SANJIAO MERIDIAN FIVE SHU POINTS

Sanjiao meridian starts from the ulnar nail corner of the ring finger and ends at the head. Since it starts from the fingertip, the five shu points start with the number 1. The first three points went in order: SJ

1, SJ 2, SJ 3. The fourth and fifth points go by skipping. The fourth point is "SJ 6" around the wrist, and the fifth point is "SJ 10" around the elbow. We were starting the first point in the Yang meridians with metal. The first point we had to find was the element point. Since Sanjiao belongs to the fire element, Sj 6 point becomes the element point. The "Sj 3 point" before it is the tonification point, and the "Sj 2 point" before it is the grandmother point. The "Sj 10 point" next to the element point is the son point, and the "Sj 1 point" after that is the grandson point (Figure 84).

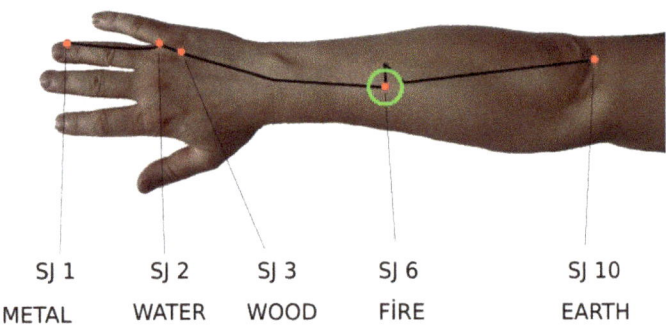

Figure 84: Sanjiao meridian five shu points

Let's say a few words about the element point "Sj 6" within the five shu points of the Sanjiao meridian. This point is a symptomatic point in the treatment of constipation. It is the most effective point in the transport of liquids among the five Shu points of the Sanjiao meridian. The fact that the organ located in the opposite direction of sanjiaon according to the organ clock is the spleen, explains the reason for this effect (Figure 85).

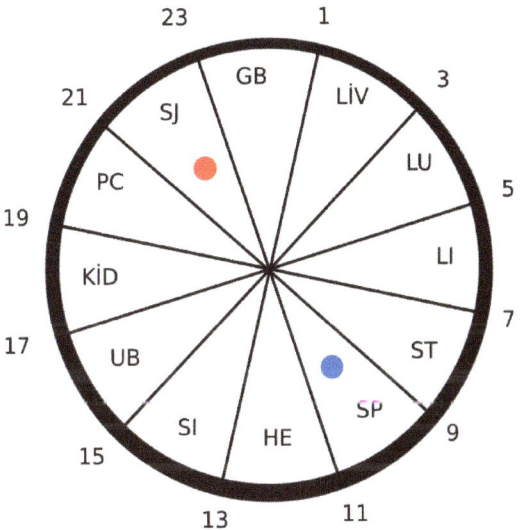

Figure 85: Sanjiao and spleen according to organ clock

CASE STUDIES RELATED TO THE ELEMENT FIRE

EXAMPLE CASE 1 (ANGINA PECTORIS):

A patient with complaints of chest pain, palpitations and numbness extending to the pinky finger of the left arm for 8-9 months, especially with exertion. On examination, the tongue corpus was thin and dry, there was a wide cleft extending anteriorly in the middle of the tongue and loss of tongue rust. The tongue apex was hyperemic. The pulse was superficial in the left distal position and was thin and tense like a wire. What should be our treatment plan in this patient?

Symptoms and examination findings indicate that the faulty pool is the heart pool. A cracked, dry, or hyperemic tongue body indicates that the pool is hot. The fact that the pulse is thin and tense like a wire indicates that the current Yin cannot control Yang and there is Yang hyperactivity (Figure 86).

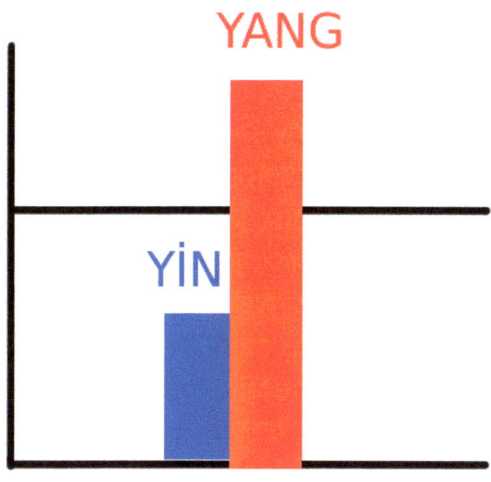

Figure 86: Yang hyperactivity due to Yin deficiency

In chronic cases where I do not find urgent intervention necessary, I am primarily in favor of turning on the cold water fountain. If the patient relaxes when the cold-water fountain is turned on, I do not sedate Yang. If not, I increase the number of cold-water fountains. If he still does not relax, I depress the Yang for a short time. Tonification points of the heart and pericardium (He 9, P 9), element points (He 8, P 8) can be used to open the cold-water fountain. Son points (SI 8, Sj 10) and grandson points (SI 1, Sj 1) through the small intestine and sanjiao meridians can be used to turn down the hot water fountain.

EXAMPLE CASE 2 (ILEUS IN THE SMALL INTESTINE):

Now I will present my own father to you as an example. The patient complained of sudden onset of nausea, vomiting, abdominal pain and occasionally made a hiccup-like sound. As a result of imaging tests, we were told that a possible hardened fecal-like structure in the small intestine obstructed the intestine and caused ileus. Tongue examination revealed clefts in the tongue corpus and dry appearance, disappearance of tongue fur in the midline and yellowing in the remaining parts (Figure 87). The patient had a weak and superficial pulse on the anterior left side.

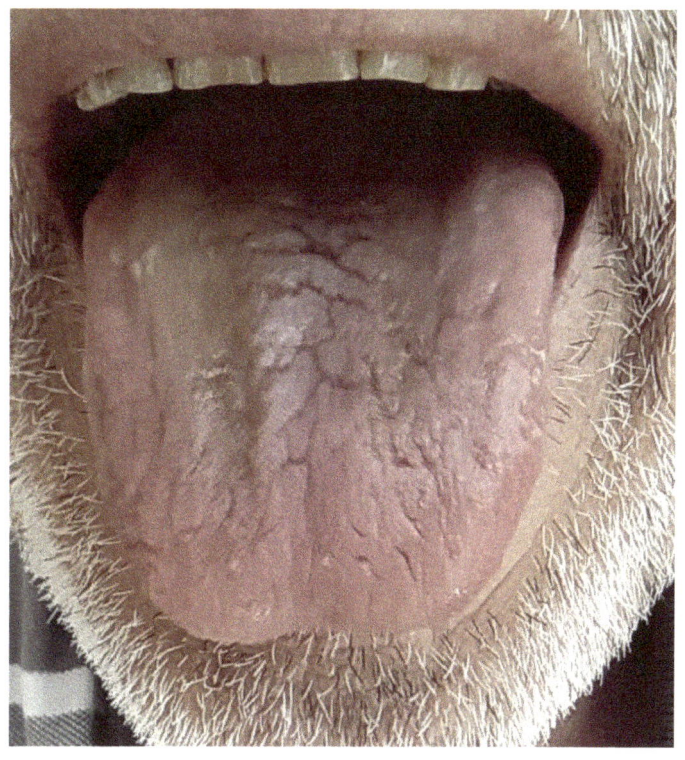

Figure 87: Tongue image

In the reference books, in cases like this one, where a defective pool is estimated, the pulse findings are recorded, especially the finding felt in the localization where that organ is represented in the pulse. So when I say that the pulse was felt weak and superficial on the anterior left side in our patient, the pulse may be felt differently in other areas, or in the same way. When you come across a pulse description like this in the source books, you will understand that the author has a possible malfunctioning pool in his/her mind and is trying to convey information to the reader about the Yin Yang state of the pool he/she is specifically targeting.

In the case study, we found the target pool with the help of Western Medicine. The language findings are in favor of Yin deficiency. The pulse also confirms this. A superficial and weak pulse indicates Yin and Yang deficiency, but Yin is much more low than Yang (Figure 88). If Yang had been normal or above normal, it would have produced a tense pulse like a wire.

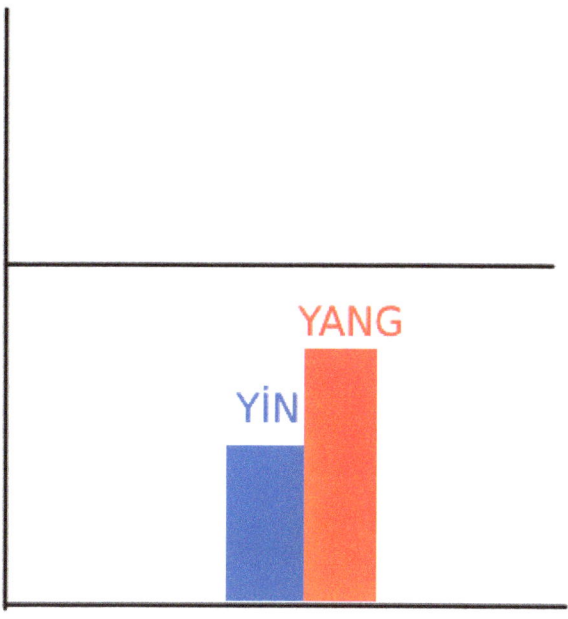

Figure 88: Empty heat

Two cold water fountains and one hot water fountain were opened in the patient. He 9 and SI 2 were used as cold water fountains and SI 3 was used as hot water fountain. Ren 4, Ren 12 and St 25 were used as local points. After 3 days of follow-up with nasogastric catheter and acupuncture, the patient's ileus picture improved and no surgical intervention was required.

In a case where the pool is hot, the logic of turning on the hot water fountain as well as the cold-water fountain may not be understood. By opening two cold water fountains and one hot water fountain, we eventually cool the pool. The small intestine is responsible for the absorption of nutrients as well as the transfer of intestinal contents to the large intestine. After the obstructive fecal content has been softened by the cold-water fountain, the intestinal contents must be delivered to the large intestine by peristaltic movements. Yang is needed for this function of the small intestine. Therefore, opening the hot water fountain will fulfill this need.

Determining deficiency and excess based on the onset of symptoms will allow you to make accurate decisions in most patients, but, as seen in this case, accepting it as the sole determining criterion can lead to misdiagnosis and ultimately incorrect treatment. For this reason, it is useful to confirm the decision of excess and deficiency based on the onset of the complaint with a tongue and pulse examination.

EXAMPLE CASE 3 (PAINFUL AFT ON TONGUE):

A patient with 1-week history of severe pain in the tongue was examined and ulcerated area in the anterior and lateral 1/3 of the tongue, hyperemia in the surrounding tissue and yellowing of the tongue rust were observed. On pulse examination, the pulse was felt as strong and superficial in the left anterior localization. What should be our treatment plan in this patient?

According to the five-element theory, certain sensory organs pointed to certain organs. Since the tongue is associated with the fire element, we thought that the defective pool was the fire element. The tongue and pulse findings confirmed this. Again, the tongue and pulse findings indicate that the pool was hot and that it was a case of excess (Figure 89). The onset of symptoms also confirmed that it was a case of excess.

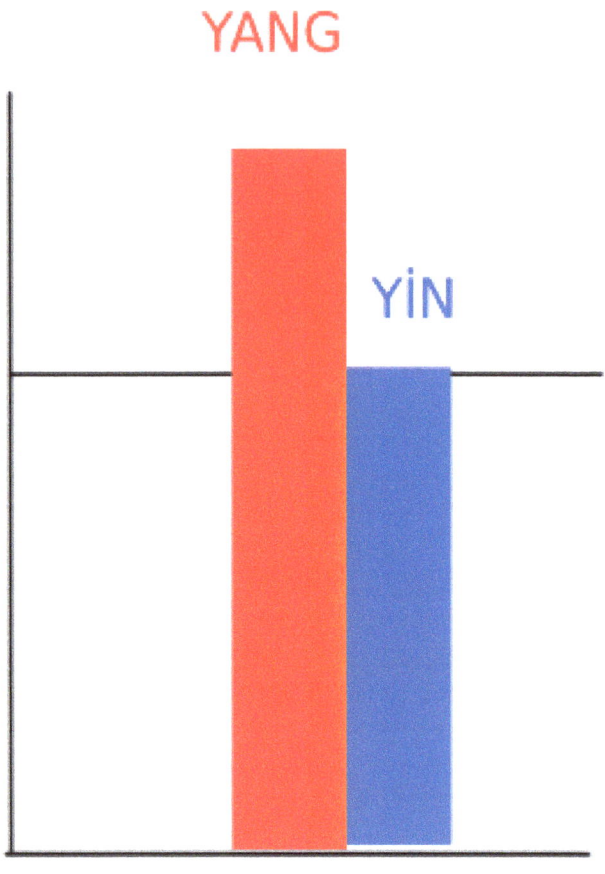

Figure 89: Full heat

We only need to turn off the hot water tap in the patient. The son points (SI 8, Sj 10) and grandson points (SI 1, Sj 1) of the small intestine and sanjiao meridians can be used for this purpose. Even if we use only the small intestine meridian, the treatment will be sufficient. In such excess cases, it is useful to do acupuncture sessions every day. Usually, 3-4 sessions are enough. As soon as the clinical picture improves, the treatment is terminated.

EXAMPLE CASE 4 (HYPERTENSION):

It was learned that the restless-looking patient, who came this morning with complaints of a feeling of heaviness in the head, imbalance, pain in the nape, and palpitations, had been suffering from hypertension for years and that these complaints recurred during hypertensive attacks. When the patient's blood pressure was examined, it was seen that it was 180/100 mmHg and his pulse was 92 beats per minute. In the tongue examination, it was observed that the tongue body appeared dry, its tip was hyperemic and there was no tongue fur. The pulse was felt as thin, tense and superficial as a string in the left anterior location. What should our treatment plan be like for the patient?

In cases of hypertension, we know from the symptoms and examination findings and author comments that the faulty pool is the fire element. Although the patient's complaints of heaviness in the head and imbalance do not indicate a specific pool, the complaint of palpitations points to the heart pool. In cases where the heart pool is heated, nape pain is often observed due to the course of the small intestine meridian. Therefore, although nape pain indicates that the faulty pool may have the fire element, it is not definitive evidence. Because the bladder meridian also passes through the nape. The fact that the patient has tachycardia, his pulse is thin, tense and superficial, especially in the left anterior position, and the tip of his tongue is hyperemic, support that the faulty pool is the fire element. Author comments also say that in hypertension, especially the heart and liver pools are the faulty pools. In cases where the liver pool becomes heated, internal wind may occur. The patient's complaint of imbalance may also be related to this. In the first chapters of the book, we said that symptoms related to hypermobility in the body bring wind to mind. This hypermobility can be objective, as in tremor, or subjective, as in vertigo. For this reason, since the liver pool is usually warm during a hypertensive attack, the left middle pulse and the left anterior pulse are often felt to be similar. Loss of tongue fur and dryness of the tongue body are signs of Yin deficiency. If the pulse findings are taken into consideration, we can say that the case is Yang hyperactivity developing on the basis of Yin deficiency (Figure 90).

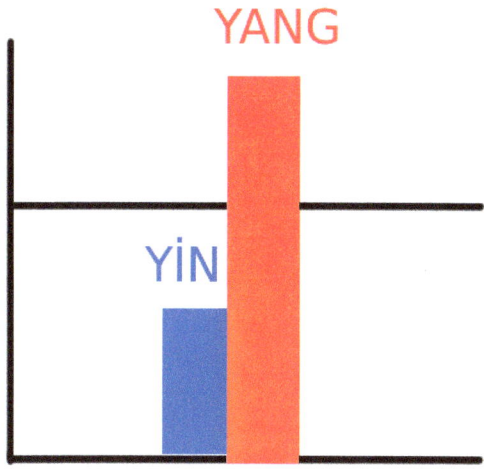

Figure 90: Yang hyperactivity due to Yin deficiency

In the light of these findings, what we should do is to turn off the hot water tap and turn on the cold water tap. In the first example, I said that in chronic cases where I don't feel that immediate intervention is necessary, I am in favor of opening the cold water fountain first, and if the patient is relieved when the cold water fountain is opened, then I don't sedate Yang. In cases like this one, where we are considering immediate intervention, I recommend closing the hot water fountain and opening the cold water fountain at the same time.

The son points (SI 8, Sj 10) and grandson points (SI 1, Sj 1) of the small intestine and sanjiao meridians can be used to turn off the hot water fountain. The tonification points (He 9, P 9) or element points (He 8, P 8) of the heart and pericardium meridians can be used to open the cold water fountain. Since the gallbladder is the organ opposite to the heart according to the organ clock, if the He 8 point is tonified, the Yang of the gallbladder will change polarity and flow into the heart as Yin energy. Thus both the Yang of the gallbladder will be reduced and the Yin of the heart will be increased.

EXAMPLE CASE 5 (CARPAL TUNNEL SYNDROME):

The patient, who had right hand wrist pain that had been disturbing enough to wake him up at night for 3-4 months, and numbness and tingling in four fingers except the little finger, was relieved by shaking, moving and rubbing his hands. On examination of the patient, who was diagnosed with carpal tunnel syndrome after EMG examination, the tongue corpus appeared swollen and pale. The pulse was felt deep, wide and soft bilaterally, especially in the anterior position. What should our treatment plan be like for the patient?

In case of complaints such as pain or numbness extending to the fingers, knowing which fingers are affected provides great convenience in finding the faulty pool. Numbness and tingling in the patient's four fingers, except the little finger, indicates all four pools. These are lung, large intestine, pericardium and sanjiao. The fact that the complaint occurs at night, the swollen and pale appearance of the tongue, and the feeling of a deep, wide and soft pulse indicate that the pool is cold. The fact that the case is in the subacute stage suggests that your Yang energy is lower than normal and your Yin energy is higher than normal (Figure 91). This is confirmed by the fact that the pulse feels deep, wide and soft.

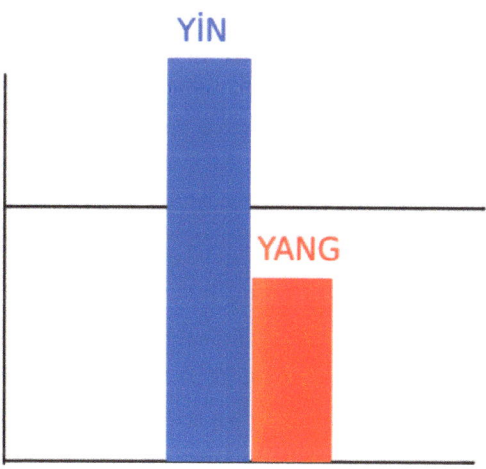

Figure 91: Yang deficiency and Yin hyperactivity

In this case, it would be appropriate to turn on the hot water fountain and turn off the cold-water fountain. We have two hot water fountains and two cold water fountains. The tonification point (Sj 3) can be used over the Sanjiao meridian, or the element point (Sj 6) with a tonifying maneuver, and the tonification point (LI 11) can be used over the large intestine meridian. Moxa can be applied to the element point (LI 1). To turn off the cold-water fountain, son and grandson points (P 7, P 5) can be used over the pericardial meridian, and son and grandson points (Lu 5, Lu 11) can be used over the lung meridian.

Even though she did not answer through the five shu points, I would like to convey here the suggestion of my esteemed teacher Radha Thambirajah for the treatment of carpal tunnel syndrome. "I think carpal tunnel syndrome is due to localized damp stagnation in the pericardial meridian. I have touched on carpal tunnel syndrome treatment in many seminars. Placing the wrist and arm flat, use 2 needles perpendicularly on the pericardial meridian (a few mm distal and proximal to the wrist crease), 2 needles lateral to the flexor carpi radialis, and 2 needles medial to the palmaris longs, for a total of 6 short needles. These will be a total of 6 needles in the wrist, all vertical, 2 in the middle and 2 on each side of the tendons. Then, we palpate the pericardial meridian starting from the distal of the arm to the proximal and needling 2 sensitive points at the distal level and 2 at the proximal level of the arm. At these 4 points, we enter the needle perpendicular to the muscle. It may also be useful to use points St 40, TW 5. After 20 minutes, remove all the needles and then apply small cupping on the wrist area and also on the palm. This is done to circulate dampness and eliminate stagnation. It will be repeated twice a week, 12 times in total. If the patient is pregnant, we may apply less treatment, we also reduce the injections and apply more local cupping. If symptoms persist after birth, more comprehensive treatment may be administered."

EXAMPLE CASE 6 (STUTTERING):

The patient, who says that he has been speaking stuttering when excited for as long as he can remember, states that he experiences pain around the navel in overly excited situations that require public speaking. On examination, it was observed that the tongue fur had disappeared, the tongue body appeared dry but there was no significant change in its color, the pulse was weak and superficial on the left side anterior, and the number of beats per minute was 88. What should our treatment plan be like for the patient?

In this case, the sensory organ, the tongue, will help us find the faulty pool. Since the tongue is a sensory organ related to the fire element and pulse findings confirm this, our target pool will be the organs belonging to the fire element. Symptoms and examination findings indicate that the pool is hot. A shallow pulse indicates that the pool is hot, and a weak pulse indicates that Yang has decreased like Yin. Likewise, the absence of tongue rust and dry tongue indicates that the pool is hot, but the absence of hyperemia on the tongue indicates that Yang is not very pronounced (Figure 92).

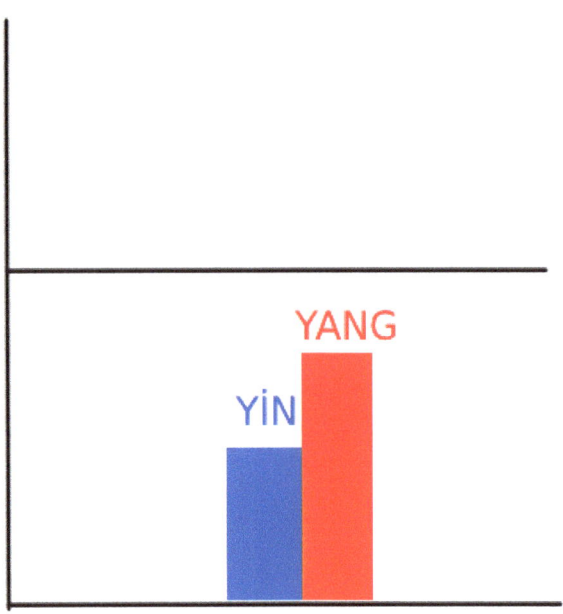

Figure 92: Empty heat

İn that case what needs to be done is to open a hot water tap along with 2-3 cold water taps. The tonification point of the heart and pericardium (He 9, P 9) and the element point of the heart (He 8) will be sufficient as a cold water tap. Of course, the element point should be used with a tonifying maneuver. The tonification point of the small intestine (SI 3) or the nene point of the heart (He 3) can be used as a hot water tap.

Sample cases can be extended further, but I think this is enough to understand the subject. Now let's move on to the wood element.

FIVE SHU POINTS OF THE LIVER MERIDIAN

The liver meridian starts from the lateral corner of the big toe and ends in the thorax. Since the starting point is the fingertip, it starts with the number 1. We said that the lung and liver follow the order. The first four points go in order: Liv 1, liv 2, liv 3 and liv 4. The fifth point is the "liv 8" point around the knee. The first point we had to find was the element point. Since the liver belongs to the wood element, the liv 1 point becomes the element point. The "liv 8 point" before it is the tonification point, and the "liv 4 point" before it is the grandmother point. The liv 2 point next to the element point is the son point, and the liv 3 point after it is the grandson point (Figure 93).

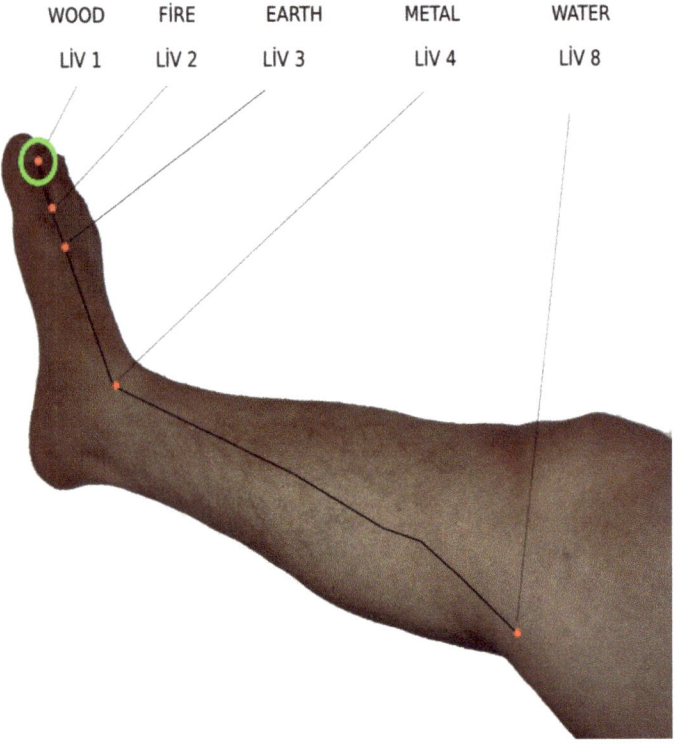

Figure 93: Five shu points on the liver meridian

Son and grandson points (liv 2, liv 3) are the points that close the tap. Since the liver meridian is the Yin meridian, of course it turns off the cold water tap. But the liv 3 point has a feature. Since the third point from the fingertip on the yin meridians is the yuan point, the liv 3 point is both the grandson point and the yuan point. For this reason, the liv 3 point has the possibility of closing the tap, as well as opening it. If we want to close the tap, we need to make our intention known with a sedating maneuver; if we want to open it, we need to make our intention known with a tonifying maneuver.

In the first chapters of our book, I said that there are many different forms of acupuncture. I said that even five element acupuncture does not have a standard practice, and that it can be applied in different ways in different schools. I would like to give an example of this through the Liv 2 point. According to the five element acupuncture we learned, we said that the son points on the Yin meridians suppress Yin to a large extent and Yang to a lesser extent. In a different five element acupuncture practice, the "Fire" points can be used to increase or decrease the Yang of the meridian. If the Yang of the meridian is to be increased, the "Fire" point is tonified; if it is to be decreased, it is sedatized. For this reason, don't be surprised if you see some sourcebooks saying, for example, "Drains liver fire, suppresses liver Yang" because liv 2 is a "Fire" point. The practitioner should act in accordance with the principles of whichever method they find more useful.

There are extra acupuncture points on the body. For example, there are bafeng extra acupuncture points between the toes. These points are used to remove wind from the body. The Liv 2 point, because it coincides with the bafeng extra acupuncture points, is mentioned among the important points that remove wind from the body.

Liv 4 point is the grandmother point of the liver meridian. The grandmother valve on the cold water fountain was flowing hot water into the pool. Since liver diseases are mostly Yang dominant diseases, this point is not used very often in practice. Hypotension is one of the indications for use. We have said that the mediocre state of emotions is not a bad thing, for example, the emotion of anger is necessary for a person to defend his rights. For this reason, Liv 4 point may come to mind for people who cannot angry and cannot defend their rights when necessary.

GALLBLADDER MERIDIAN FIVE SHU POINTS

The gallbladder meridian starts from the head and ends at the lateral corner of the fourth toe. The point where it ends at the foot is GB 44. While the first three points go in order in all meridians, we said that the gallbladder meridian is an exception. On the gallbladder meridian, the first two points follow the order, the third, fourth and fifth points do not follow the order. The points are GB 44, GB 43, GB 41, GB 38 and GB 34 respectively. Now let's do the naming. Yang meridians started with metal. GB 44 is called metal, GB 43 is called water, GB 41 is called wood, GB 38 is called fire, GB 34 is called earth. The first point we would find was the element point. In this case, GB 41 point is the element point. The one before the element point is the tonification point (GB 43), and the one before it is the grandmother point (GB 44). The point after the element point is the son point (GB 38), and the point after the son point is the grandson point (GB 34) (Figure 94).

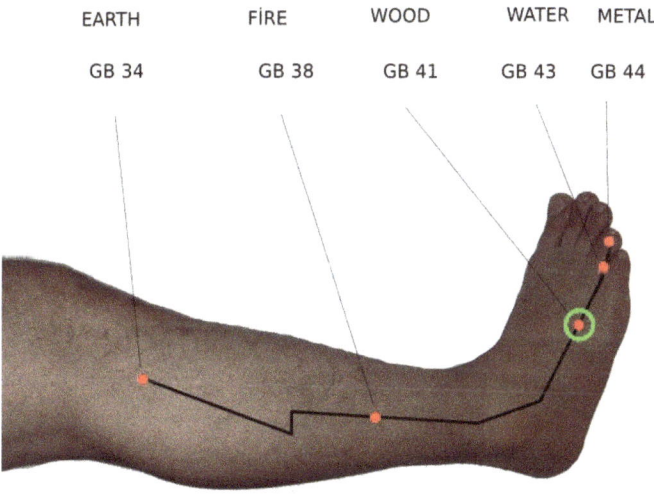

Figure 94: Five shu points on the gallbladder meridian

The point GB 41 is not only the element point of the meridian but also the confluent point of the Dai Mai meridian, one of the unusual meridians. As we said before, if we want to send a warning to the extraordinary meridian, we need to use an additional point. Since this is not the subject of five element acupuncture, let's stop here. If we want to close the tap with the element point "GB 41" of the meridian, we must perform a sedating maneuver, and if we want to open it, we must perform a tonifying maneuver. Since tree pool diseases are more Yang dominant, the point is usually used with a sedating maneuver. When sedated, Yang energy changes polarity and flows as Yin energy to the heart in the opposite direction according to the organ clock (Figure 95).

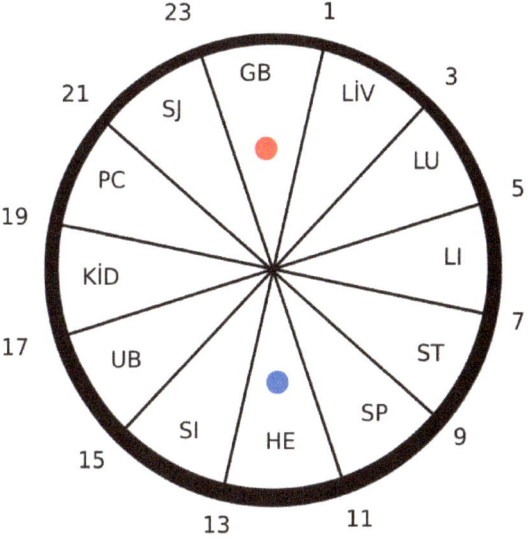

Figure 95: Organ clock

GB 43 is the point that opens the faucet. Just like the liv 2 point, it is among the wind elimination points because it coincides with the bafeng extra acupuncture points between the fingers. If we want to use it for wind elimination, the point should be used with a sedating maneuver.

Gb 34 point is the point that closes the tap as it is the grandson point, as well as the effective point of muscles and tendons. Therefore, it can be used in all locomotor system diseases.

SAMPLE CASES ABOUT THE WOOD ELEMENT

EXAMPLE CASE 1 (MIGRINE):

The patient described severe headache attacks that recurred once or twice a week for 3-4 years, hitting both sides of the temples and occasionally behind the eyes. Before the attack, he complained of lightening in the eyes and nausea. The patient had severe pain during the examination. During the examination, it was observed that the tongue body was thin and dry, hyperemic on the right lateral side, there were clefts in places, and there was no tongue rust. The pulse was felt as thin and tense, especially in the left middle localization. What should our treatment plan be like for the patient?

In patients who describe their pain as a specific area rather than a meridian course, if you can find the possible pool according to sensitive points by palpation, you can only perform the treatment on the meridian of that pool. For a migraine patient, as in the example, the hot pool is usually a tree pool. If you are not sure if it is the gallbladder meridian by palpation of tender points, also use the sanjiao meridian in the treatment.

In diseases with recurrent attacks, we expect to see one of the Yin and Yang energies increased and the other decreased during the attack. The patient's tongue and pulse findings show that the pool is hot. Therefore, we expect Yang to increase and Yin to decrease. Loss of tongue fur, cracks in the tongue, thin pulse indicate Yin deficiency, and hyperemic corpus and tense pulse indicate Yang hyperactivity (Figure 96).

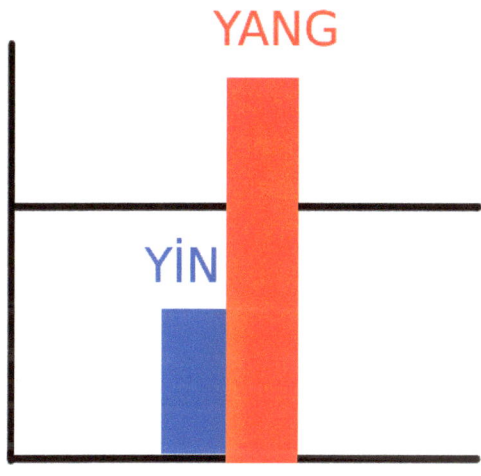

Figure 96: Yang hyperactivity due to Yin deficiency

In light of these findings, you should turn off the hot water tap and turn on the cold water tap in the patient. You can use the son and grandson points (GB 38, GB 34) on the gallbladder meridian to turn off the hot water tap. As you master the subject, as you gain mastery in this work, if you contemplate on which organ you are directing the energy towards with the points you turn off the tap, your success rates in treatment will increase much more. For example, if you close the tap on this patient with point GB 38, since this point is the "Fire" point, it will send the energy to the fire element. Let's suppose that symptoms such as palpitations, insomnia and tongue and pulse findings indicate that the fire pool is hot in this patient, instead of directing Yang energy to the fire element through the GB 38 point, you direct it to the earth element through the GB 34 point. In such a patient, the result of using the GB 34 point will be more favorable than the result of using the GB 38 point. If you close the hot water tap on the gallbladder through the element point (GB 41), then the result you will get from the treatment will be at the highest level. This is because, as we said above, according to the organ clock, the organ in the opposite direction to the gallbladder is the heart. If the GB 41 point is sedated, the Yang energy in the gallbladder changes polarity and flows into the heart as Yin energy. Thus, both the wood pool and the fire pool will be cooled.

As you can see, five element acupuncture is the art of balancing energy. You can direct the energy to any organ you want. Of course, this kind of comprehensive thinking requires the knowledge of which point and which organ the energy is directed to and the ability to evaluate the Yin Yang balance in the organs, which is the result of a certain amount of time and patience.

The tonification point (Liv 8), the element point (Liv 1) over the liver meridian, and the grandmother point (GB 44) over the gallbladder meridian can be used to turn on the cold water fountain. You can also use Liv 3 points with a tonifying maneuver. I have previously suggested that in chronic cases with recurrent attacks, you should first turn on the cold water fountain, and if the patient does not feel relieved, add the second cold water fountain. You can do the same thing in this case. First of all, you turn on 1-2 cold water fountains, or even a third cold water fountain if necessary, and if it does not provide relief, you turn off the hot water fountain. As far as I have observed, it is generally necessary to turn off the hot water fountain in migraine patients during an attack.

Hyperemia on the lateral side of the tongue, which occurs during an attack in migraine patients, usually regresses rapidly after the attack. During the inter-attack period, as Yang hyperactivity disappears, the tense pulse also disappears. If the pulse is weak and superficial during the patient's pain-free period, the Yin Yang diagram expected in the patient is as shown in figure 97. In this case, 2-3 cold water fountains and 1 hot water fountain are opened during the treatment.

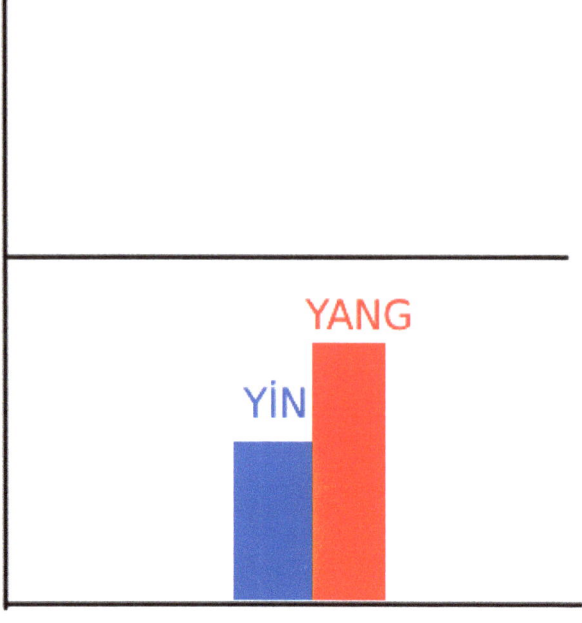

Figure 97: Empty hot

If the pulse is still tense and superficial during the patient's pain-free period, although not as much as during the attack, the Yin Yang diagram expected in the patient is as shown in figure 98. In this case, only 2-3 cold water fountains are opened during the treatment. Of course, this is not always easy to distinguish. If you cannot differentiate and if the patient's pain is triggered when you turn on 2-3 cold water fountains as well as 1 hot water fountain, you stop the process of turning on the hot water fountain.

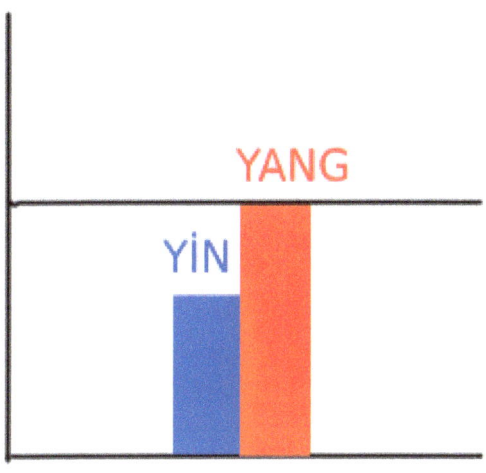

Figure 98: Empty hot

EXAMPLE CASE 2 (ACUTE CHOLECYSTITIS):

The patient's complaint, which describes pain in the right-sided hypochondriac area, started suddenly last night. The patient, who had complaints of nausea, loss of appetite and abdominal bloating, underwent ultrasound and detected gallbladder stones and mucosal thickening compatible with cholecystitis. The patient's slippery pulse was detected in the middle-left wrist, and the tongue fur was observed to be thick and yellow, and the lateral part of the tongue body was hyperemic.

We have utilized examination findings and Western Medicine imaging to identify the defective pool. When describing the methods of finding the defective pool, we said that the area of complaint guides us. We said to be careful with pain in the abdomen and thorax where the internal organs are located, and that organ diseases can cause pain at the front mu and back shu points. The case of cholecystitis is a good example to illustrate our point. If you say that the hypochondriac area is in the anterior part of the body and you use the meridians in the anterior part of the extremities for treatment, you are wrong. Giovanni Macciocia, quoting from "The Spiritual Axis", says that hypochondriac pain is always associated with the liver and gall bladder.

A hyperemic tongue corpus and yellowing of the tongue fur indicate that the pool is hot, and thickened tongue fur and a slippery pulse are evidence of dampness as well as an increase in heat. Also author interpretations interpret cases of cholecystitis as damp-heat in the gallbladder (Figure 99).

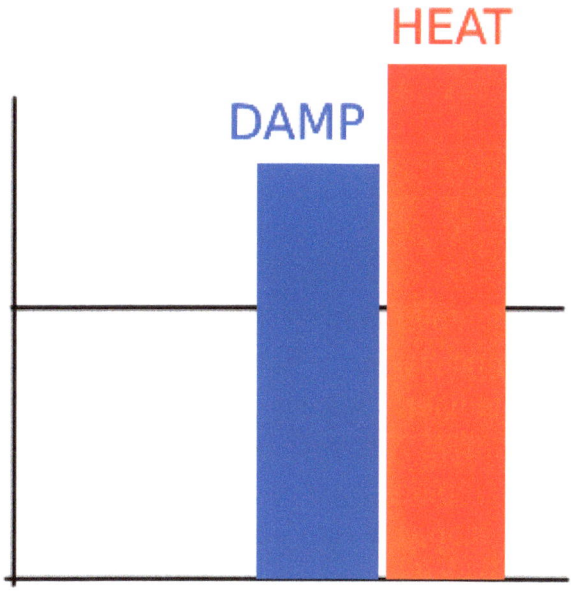

Figure 99: Damp heat

Earlier we said that in cases of damp heat there is both Yin and Yang increase, just like in cases of phlegm, the difference being that in damp heat Yang is the first cause and Yin increase is in response. Therefore, in these cases, either the hot water tap is turned off alone or both hot and cold water taps are turned off together.

The son and grandson points of the gallbladder meridian (GB 38, GB 34) can be used to turn off the hot water tap, and the son and grandson points of the liver meridian (liv 2, liv 3) can be used to turn off the cold water tap. The front mu point of the gallbladder (GB 24) can also be used as a local point.

EXAMPLE CASE 3 (EPILEPSY):

It was learned that the patient, who had epileptic attacks occasionally for 5-6 years, usually had a quick temper, occasionally had epistaxis after hypertensive attacks, and twice had Achilles tendon rupture after a medium speed run. On examination, the eye was hyperemic, the tongue corpus was thin and dry, and there were cracks on the lateral side. The pulse was weak and superficial, especially in the left middle localization. What should be our treatment plan in this patient?

In the first chapters of the book, we said that the presence of wind is suspected in diseases and symptoms such as convulsions, tics, and tremor, which progress with excessive activity in the body. If internal wind, accompanying symptoms, tongue and pulse findings support it, it directs us to the liver as the faulty pool. The liver is the cause of physiological internal wind. In liver Yin deficiency, liver fire and liver blood deficiency, physiological internal wind can turn into pathological internal wind and internal wind symptoms and signs may occur. When we say inner wind, you will understand pathological inner wind unless we add any explanatory information. It's easy to understand why internal wind appears when the liver pool heats up. To understand this, we gave an example of the air flow that occurs upwards from the chimney when the fireplace is lit. It is not easy to understand why internal wind symptoms occur in liver blood deficiency. To make this easier to understand, Giovanni gives the analogy of wind emerging between large underground spaces in metro stations. This simile, as he stated, can be understood as meaning that the wind fills the gap in the blood vessels in case of blood deficiency. Although this explanation does not seem very satisfactory to me personally, I thought it appropriate to convey it to the reader in case it helps to understand the subject. Cases of blood deficiency may be reflected in the clinic with hot pool symptoms and signs, as well as cold pool symptoms and signs. My personal opinion is that liver blood failure cases with hot pool symptoms cause internal wind.

The faulty pool is wood pool. The patient's eyes being hyperemic, the tongue corpus being thin, dry and cracked, and the pulse being superficial are signs that the pool is hot. If the pulse was shallow and tense, it would indicate that Yang was normal or higher than normal. Being superficial and weak indicates a hot pool where Yang is also low. During the attack, Yin cannot control Yang and Yang hyperactivity occurs. If we had seen the patient during this period, we would have seen his pulse as likely superficial, thin and wire-like. After the attack, the Yin Yang appearance returns to its previous state (Figure 100).

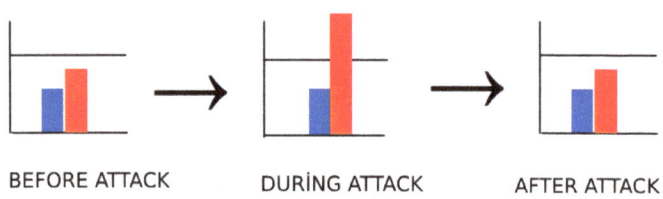

Figure 100: Yin Yang image of the patient before, during and after the attack

In light of these findings, what we need to do in this patient we see between attacks is to open 2-3 cold water taps and one hot water tap. If you are afraid that an attack will occur if the hot water tap is opened, you can only turn on the cold water tap for a while and postpone this process until the next sessions.

The tonification point (Liv 8), the element point (Liv 1) over the liver meridian, and the nene point (GB 44) over the gallbladder meridian can be used to turn on the cold water fountain. You can also use Liv 3 points with a tonifying maneuver. You can use the hot water fountain over the tonification point of the gallbladder meridian (GB 43). The element point (GB 41) with a tonifying maneuver or the grandmother point of the liver meridian (Liv 4) are among the points that can be used for this purpose.

It would be better if wind elimination points are also added to the treatment. By the way, let's also tell you which points are used for wind elimination. Radha Thambirajah has conveyed these points neatly in his book. I am quoting from him and passing it on to you below.

-GB 20 and Du 16: Head and neck

-SI 12: Shoulder and arm

-UB 12: Back, Lung

-GB 31: Hip and leg

-Ba Feng: These are the extra acupuncture points between the toes. These are four in each leg, eight in total. Although these points eliminate the wind in the feet, one of them, Liv 2 point, is the wind elimination point for the whole body.

-Ba Xie: These are the extra acupuncture points between the fingers. These are eight in number, just like the ones on the feet, and they take the wind away from the hand.

EXAMPLE CASE 4 (VERTIGO):

The patient, who had been complaining of occasional dizziness for 3-4 years, started to experience dizziness again in the last two weeks. No hearing loss, no tinnitus. The patient states that he gets tired very quickly and that his complaints increase especially after intense work and stress. She also states that her complaints intensify during and after her menstrual period, and that her periods are long and insufficient in quantity. On tongue examination, the tongue body is pale, especially more prominent in the lateral areas. A shallow cleft was observed in the lateral and midline of the tongue (Figure 101). During pulse examination, we felt the left middle pulse as thin, weak and superficial. What should our treatment plan be like for the patient?

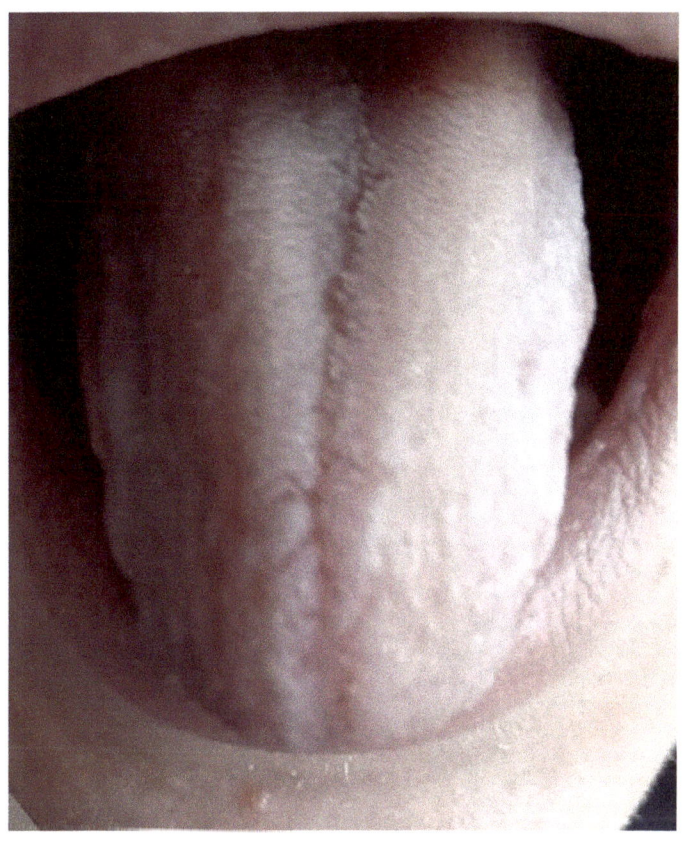

Figure 101: Tongue image

First, we will need to find the faulty pool in the patient. In the presence of internal wind symptoms, the first pool we should turn to is the liver pool. In cases of hypermobility, internal wind came to mind. This hypermobility can be objective or subjective, as in vertigo. Pale tongue appearance occurs due to Yang deficiency or blood deficiency. If there is yang deficiency, the tongue will be swollen, pale and moist. In case of blood deficiency, the tongue becomes thin, dry and pale. Although this patient's tongue does not appear to be thin, it is more appropriate to diagnose blood deficiency. It is impossible to have Yang deficiency, in fact, the cleft in the tongue indicates that there is Yin deficiency. In some patients, everything may not be as we expect. Source books say that the tongue becomes thin in case of blood deficiency, but sometimes a thick tongue may appear as in this patient. The reason for this is likely that damp accumulation has occurred in the patient secondary to stomach-spleen Yin deficiency, as can be understood from the cleft in the middle of the tongue. Blood deficiency may appear with hot pool symptoms in some cases, and with cold pool symptoms in some patients. In this patient, the dry and cracked structure of the tongue and the superficial pulse indicate that the pool is hot (Figure 102).

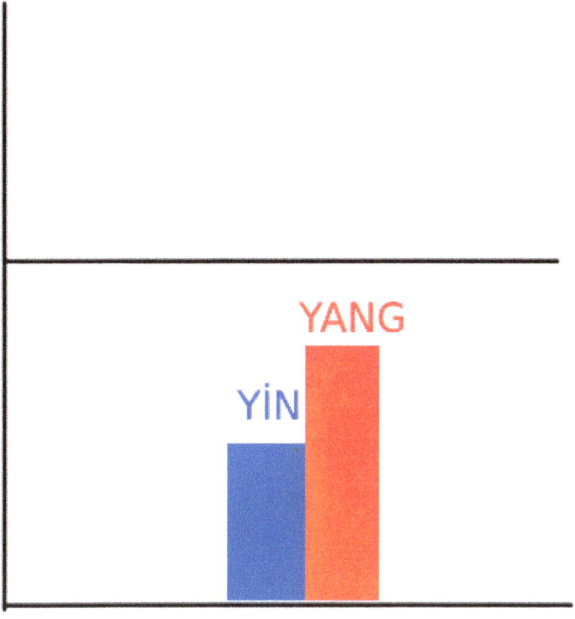

Figure 102: Empty hot

In light of these findings, it would be appropriate to open 2-3 cold water fountains and one hot water fountain on the wood element, as well as use blood-forming points.

As we said in the previous example, the tonification point (Liv 8), the element point (Liv 1) over the liver meridian and the grandmother point (GB 44) over the gallbladder meridian can be used to turn on the cold water fountain. Also, Liv 3 point can also be used with a tonifying maneuver. You can use the hot water fountain over the tonification point of the gallbladder meridian (GB 43). The element point (GB 41) with a tonifying maneuver or the grandmother point of the liver meridian (Liv 4) are among the points that can be used for this purpose.

In order to understand the points that increase blood formation, it is useful to know how blood is formed according to TCM. "Gu Qi" coming from the spleen combines with "Yuan Qi" coming from the kidney and turns into blood in the heart (Figure 103). Although some sources include "Air Qi" coming from the lungs, the heart, kidney and spleen meridians are generally used in blood production. The patient's cleft in the middle of the tongue already tells us to nourish the spleen Yin. For this purpose, spleen tonification point (Sp 2) or element point (Sp 3) can be used. Likewise, 2-3 cold water fountains and one hot water fountain can be used through these organs. The element point of the stomach (St 36) is also suitable as a hot water fountain. Although the kidney meridian will be explained in the next topic, the element point (Kid 10), the tonification point (Kid 7) can be used as a cold water fountain, and the grandmother point of the kidney (Kid 3) can be used as a hot water fountain. According to TCM, since blood is formed within the heart, Thambirajah uses points on the heart in all kinds of blood deficiency cases, whether heart blood deficiency or liver blood deficiency. The tonification point of the heart (He 9), the element point (He 8) can be used as a cold water fountain over the heart, and the grandmother point of the heart (He 3) can be used as a hot water fountain.

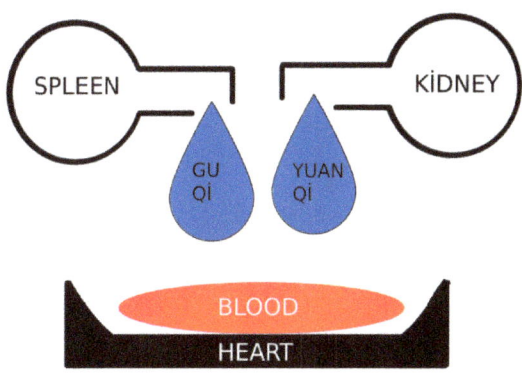

Figure 103: Formation of blood

Although not among the five shu points, but because it is relevant, let me also mention the additional points used in blood production. Among the eight influential points, the influential point of the marrow (GB 39), the influential point of the blood (UB 17), and the influential point of the bone (UB 11) are also points used in blood production.

EXAMPLE CASE 5 (VERTIGO AND WAIST PAIN):

The patient had severe dizziness for about 10 days. He had this dizziness for 5-6 years and it recurred occasionally. The patient also had lower back pain, and his pain increased with movement throughout the day. On examination, the tongue body of the patient, who had stage 1 nystagmus tapping to the left, appeared slightly dry, but no obvious pathological findings were observed (Figure 104). The pulse was generally felt as superficial and partially tense in all locations. What should our treatment plan be like for the patient?

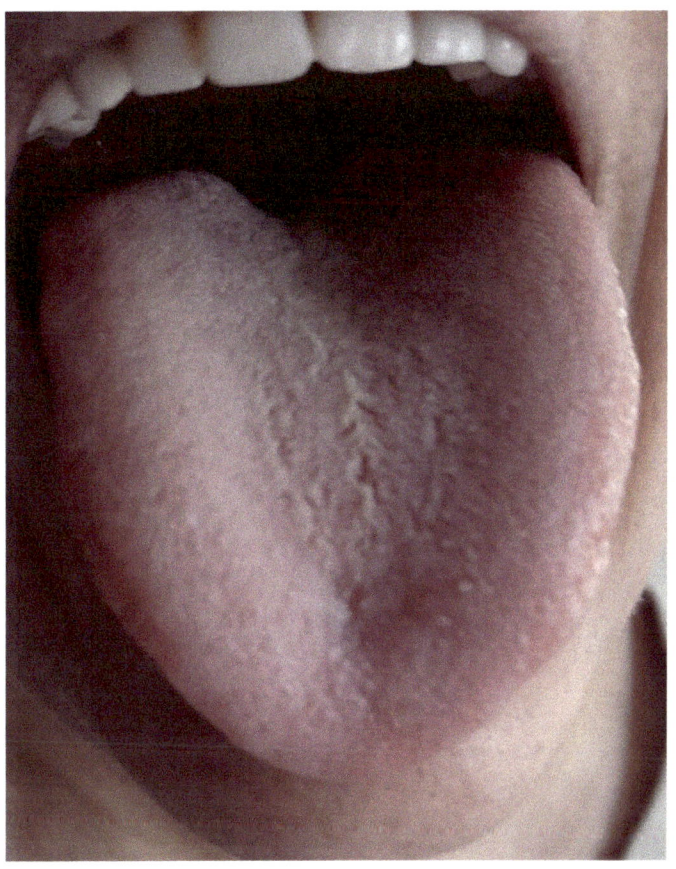

Figure 104: Tongue image

As I explained in the previous example, since vertigo is considered as internal wind, it primarily directs us to the liver as the faulty pool. In some cases, you may not encounter any findings in the language that will guide you. As in this patient, the pulse may not indicate a specific pool. In this case, the symptoms will be the determining factor in finding the faulty pool. Tongue and pulse findings tell us that the pool is warm. Interestingly, this patient is a patient who states that she does not like going to the hairdresser at all, that the hair dryer drives her crazy, that her complaints increase significantly in windy weather, and that she does not like noise and light at all. These symptoms also support the presence of hot wind. The patient's complaint of low back pain was not his primary presenting complaint. The pain he described was a Yang dominant pain. The water element is the mother of the wood element. This case is a good example of cases where the mother cannot feed her son. The Yin Yang diagram we expect in the patient is as follows (Figure 105).

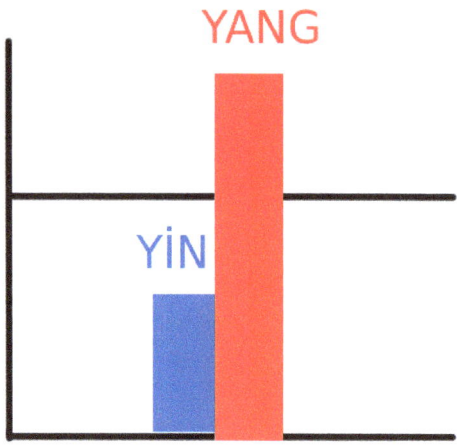

Figure 105: Yang hyperactivity due to Yin deficiency

I used the Yin nourishing points on both the kidney and liver meridian. I also added points to remove the wind. I used the tonification point (Liv 8) and the yuan point with tonifying maneuver (Liv 3) on the liver meridian, the element point (Kid 10) with tonifying maneuver and the tonification point (Kid 7) on the kidney meridian. I used the GB 20 and Liv 2 points to remove the wind. The patient felt great relief in the first session. Her nystagmus disappeared. After the second session the next day, the dizziness was completely resolved. I would like to draw the reader's attention. See, in this patient there was no need to sedate Yang at all. If she had not relaxed with the Yin tonification, I would have had to sedate Yang as well.

EXAMPLE CASE 6 (MIGRAINE AND ANKLE TENDON RUPTURE)

The patient described severe headache attacks on the left side of the head for 5-6 years, recurring once or twice a week, occasionally extending to the back of the eyes and the top of the head, and this pain increased with light and noise. Tendon rupture was diagnosed in the patient who had right ankle pain radiating to the leg for about 3 years. The patient's ankle pain was triggered by cold. Especially when the vehicle air conditioner was directed to the foot, the pain became very pronounced. On examination, it was determined that the pain extending from the ankle to the leg and foot dorsum followed the gallbladder meridian. Tongue examination revealed a thin and partially dry tongue corpus. Tongue fur was interpreted as partially thick, dry and white in colour (Figure 106). The patient's pulse was felt as superficial, thin and partially tense in the left central localisation. What should be our treatment plan in this patient?

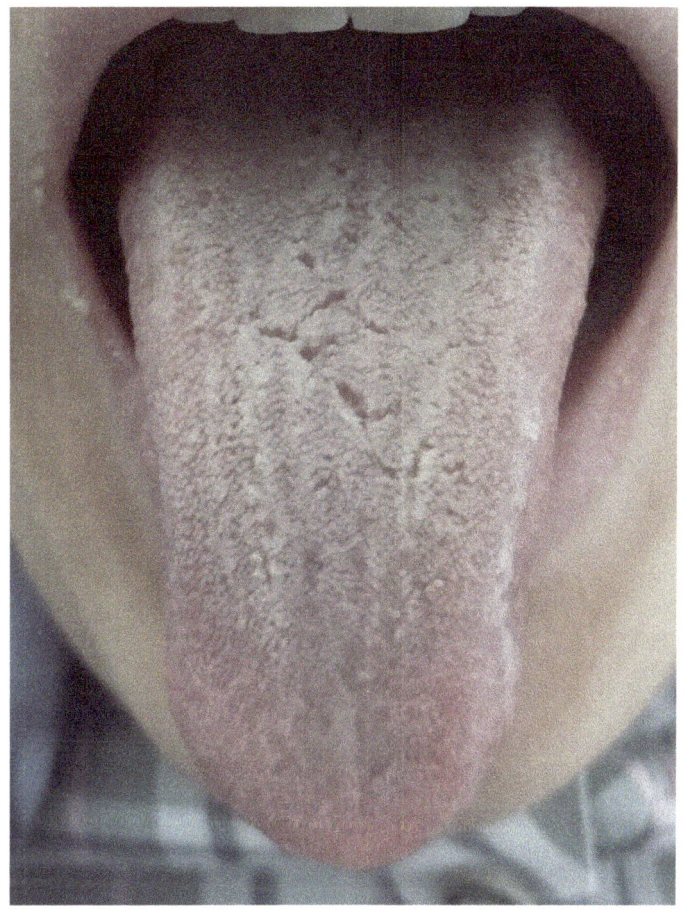

Figure 106: Tongue image

From the meridian course, we understand that the faulty pool is the gallbladder meridian. This case is a very interesting case. While the patient describes a Yang dominant pain in the head, he describes a Yin dominant pain in the foot. In such cases, Yin and Yang are thought to be close to each other. For this reason, pain on the Yang side of the body, such as the head, may be Yang dominant, while on the Yin side of the body, such as the foot, it may be Yin dominant. Considering the patient's pulse, it is understood that Yin and Yang decrease together, but Yang is partially dominant compared to Yin (Figure 107)

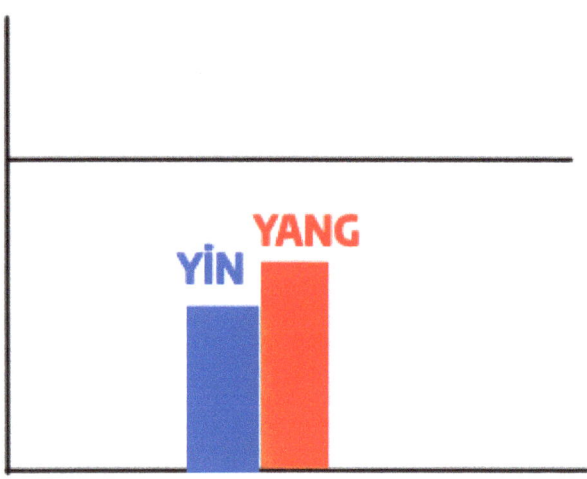

Figure 107: Yin and Yang reduction with Yang dominant

In such chronic cases, it is necessary to focus on the body of the tongue rather than the tongue fur. In chronic cases where the tongue fur is thick and dry like this, more constipation is expected, and we confirmed that constipation was present when we questioned.

In this type of case, if we say that there is a Yang dominant headache and suppress Yang and feed Yin, we will see that the foot pain is exacerbated. Therefore, what we need to do is to open 2 cold water fountains and one hot water fountain. The tonification point of the liver (Liv 8) and the yuan point with tonifying manoeuvre (Liv 3) can be used to open the cold water fountain, and the tonification point of the gallbladder (GB 43) can be used to open the hot water fountain. Although we have not yet seen the long-term results of this patient, his complaints were relieved after only the second acupuncture session.

The examples can be extended further, but since our aim is to give the reader the practice of approaching patients on the principles we have explained in the shortest time possible, let's assume that the examples of the wood element are sufficient and continue with the water element.

KIDNEY MERIDIAN FIVE SHU POINTS

The kidney meridian starts from the sole of the foot and ends in the thorax. Since its starting point is the sole of the foot, it starts with the number 1. The first three points go in order: Kid 1, kid 2, kid 3. The fourth and fifth points go by skipping, the fourth point is "kid 7" around the ankle, the fifth point is "kid 10" around the knee. The first point we had to find was the element point. Kidney Since it belongs to the water element, it becomes the "Kid 10" element point. The one before it is the "Kid 7" tonification point, and the one before it is the "Kid 3" grandmother point. The "Kid 1" point next to the element point is the son point, and the "Kid 2" point after that is the grandchild point (Figure 108)

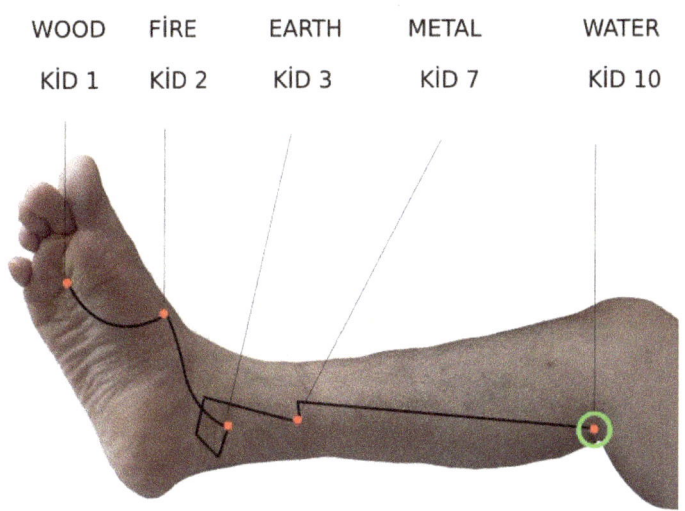

Figure 108: Kidney meridian five shu points

Since the kidney meridian is the only meridian that reaches the sole of the foot, diseases related to the sole and heel are treated through the kidney meridian. Kid 1 and kid 2 points are the points that close the tap. I think it goes without saying that you turn off the cold water tap because it is a Yin meridian. Since one of the tissues associated with the water element is bone tissue, it is not recommended to use kid 1 and kid 2 points in growing children due to the possibility of causing growth and development retardation. It is also not recommended for use in the elderly with osteoporosis and bone fractures during the healing period. Kid 1 point can be used as an emergency point in cases of epileptic attacks, seizures due to fever, or fainting.

Kid 3 point is a featured point. The third point from the distal in the yin meridians was the yuan point. Since this point is a yuan point, it has the potential to increase the Yin of the kidney, and since it is a grandmother point, it also has the potential to increase the Yang of the kidney. For this reason, it can be used for both Yin deficiencies and Yang deficiencies of the kidney.

You can also witness that there is a constant debate in the sources about the Kid 7 point. According to some sources, it increases the Yang of the kidney, and according to some sources, it increases the Yin of the kidney. This is partly due to the fact that five element acupuncture is applied in different ways among different schools. According to the five element acupuncture we have learned, it increases the Yin and partially the Yang of the kidney. That's why we say it is the point that turns on the cold water fountain.

BLADDER MERIDIAN FIVE SHU POINTS

The bladder meridian starts from the head and ends at the lateral corner of the little toe. The point where it ends at the foot is UB 67 point. The first three points go in order: UB 67, UB 66, UB 65. The fourth and fifth points go by skipping, the fourth point is UB 60 at the ankle, the fifth point is UB 40 behind the knee. Now let's do the naming. Yang meridians started with metal. UB 67 is called metal, UB 66 is called water, UB 65 is called wood, UB 60 is called fire, UB 40 is called earth. The first point we would find was the element point. In this case UB 66 is the element point. The one before the element point (UB 67) is the tonification point, and the one before it (UB 40) is the grandmother point. The point after the element point (UB 65) is the son point, and the point after that (UB 60) is the grandson point (Figure 109).

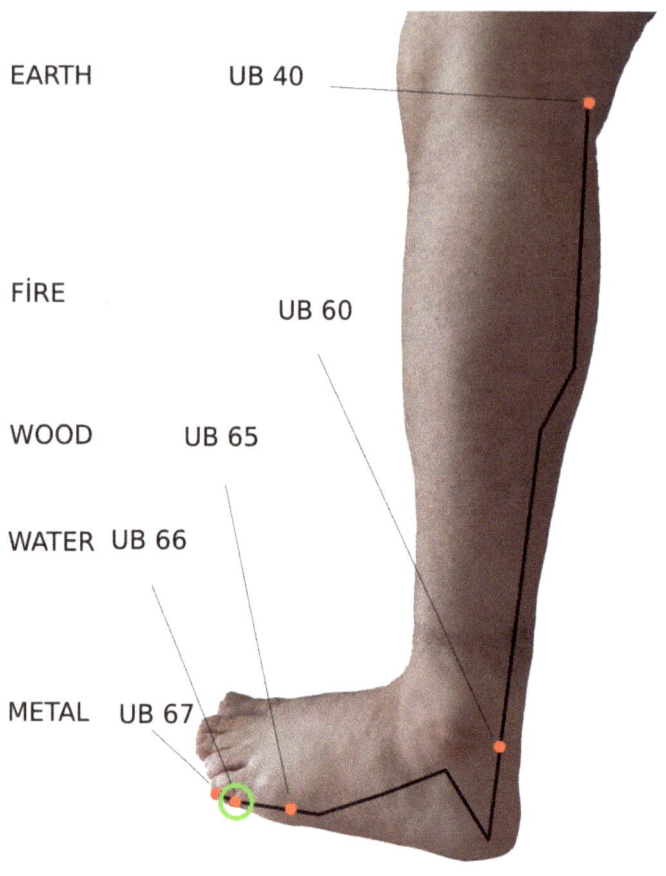

Figure 109: Five shu points of the bladder meridian

UB 67 point is the point that opens the tap. It greatly increases the Yang of the bladder and indirectly the kidney. The uterus and prostate do not have their own meridians. Diseases related to these are treated through the bladder meridian. Since the UB

67 point also increases the Yang of the uterus, it increases uterine contractions in that area. Therefore, its use is contraindicated without a specific purpose such as fetal malposition and delay in birth. Applying moxa to the UB 67 point in babies with breech presentation is an effective treatment method frequently used in clinics to position the baby in a head-down position.

UB 65 and UB 60 points are the points that close the tap. UB 60 point is frequently used both as a local point and as a point that balances energy in Achilles tendinitis. Again, UB 60 point is preferred rather than UB 65 point in the treatment of Yang dominant neck pain. This may be due to the effect of Master Tung acupuncture. In Master Tung acupuncture, the point is selected by taking advantage of the anatomical similarity between the limbs and the body. For example, since the wrist and ankle are anatomically similar to the neck region of the human body, choosing points from this region for neck pain is one of the treatment principles of this method.

UB 40 point is the grandmother point and increases the Yin of the bladder. Giovanni states that he does not prefer the UB 40 point for Yin dominant back pain. However, point UB 40 is used as the empirical distal point for the waist. Giovanni does not practice five element acupuncture and makes this suggestion as a result of his own practical practices and based on his experiences. The five element acupuncture we learned confirms Giovanni's experience and explains why very well, as you can see.

SAMPLE CASES ABOUT THE WATER ELEMENT

EXAMPLE CASE1 (BACK PAIN):

The patient had been complaining of severe lower back pain hitting the back of the leg for a week. The pain was very severe when he woke up in the morning. It increased when he started to move, but it decreased with movement during the day. The pain felt stabbing, especially in situations that required bending forward, such as brushing teeth or washing the face. When questioned, it was learned that his urine was abundant and light in colour. He stated that he had a history of such painful attacks from time to time before. When the pain localization to the leg was palpated, several tender points were detected along the bladder meridian. The tongue body was observed to be swollen and pale, and tooth marks were visible. The tongue fur was partially thick and white in color. The pulse was felt as deep, broad and soft in consistency at the proximal and mid-level on the right side. What should our treatment plan be like for the patient?

In this case, it is obvious that the faulty pool is the bladder meridian. Therefore, let's try to directly interpret the second step. So let's find out whether the pool is hot or cold. The fact that the patient's complaints decrease with movement during the day indicates that the pool is cold. We said that attention should be paid to damp pain. We stated that they experience stiffness when they wake up in the morning, therefore the first movement is very painful, and with this feature, they may be mistakenly diagnosed as Yang dominant pain. Although damp-type pains increase in the first few hours at the beginning of movement, they begin to relieve during the day, with movement and as the body warms up. So, this made us think that the pool was cold. These patients often state that their pain becomes stabbing during activities that require bending forward, as stated in the history. Since the front side is Yin, leaning forward can make the Yin of these patients more prominent and cause pain. This story also supports that the pool is cool. Tongue and pulse findings also confirm that the pool is cool. Since the event is chronic and recurrent and the patient comes to us during an attack, we expect to see one of the Yin and Yang energies increased and the other decreased. Since we found the pool to be cold, we interpret the Yin energy as increased and the Yang energy as decreased (Figure 110).

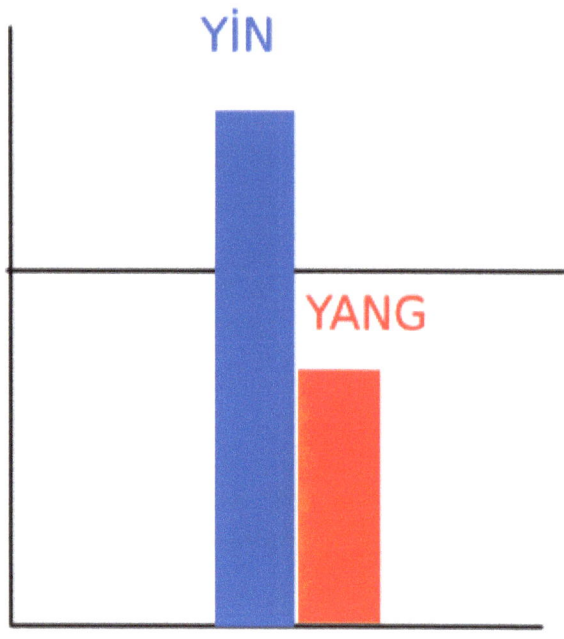

Figure 110: Yang deficiency, Yin hyperactivity

In this case, what we need to do is to turn off the cold water fountain and turn on the hot water fountain. I have said that I consider sedation as a secondary concern in chronic recurrent cases. In this case, first 2-3 hot water fountains are turned on, and if the patient does not feel relieved, the cold water fountain is turned off. The tonification point of the bladder meridian (UB 67) or the element point (UB 66) with a tonifying maneuver or the grandmother point of the kidney meridian (Kid 3) can be used to turn on the hot water fountain. The son (Kid 1) and grandson (Kid 2) points of the kidney meridian can be used to cover the cold water. It would also be appropriate to use points that remove dampness from the earth element in the patient. Although Sp 9 (lasix point) first comes to mind for this purpose, this point is not very suitable for this case as it sends Yin energy to the kidney and will further increase the Yin Load of the kidney. It would be appropriate to add the St 40 point, which is the luo point of the stomach, known as the expectorant point, to the treatment. Actually, I wasn't thinking much about talking about points other than the five shu points in this book, but I came to the conclusion that it would be appropriate to briefly talk about luo yuan point combinations.

Between two conjugate meridians there are luo channels through which energy can pass into each other. If we want energy transfer through this luo channel, if we use the luo point on one of the Yin Yang pair channels, we need to use the yuan point on the other. There is disagreement in the sources as to whether the energy passes from the luo point to the yuan point or from the yuan point towards the luo point. You can perform this operation on both points. If you want the energy to be transferred from the luo point to the yuan point, the luo point is sedated and the yuan point is tonified. If you want the energy to be transferred from the yuan point to the luo point, the yuan point is sedated and the luo point is tonified. Luo yuan point combinations are frequently used in treatment in cases where one of the Yin and Yang energies decreases and the other increases, as in our example case. Let's explain the use of these points a little on our example case. In our example case where we want to reduce the Yin and increase the Yang of the kidney, we do this in two ways through luo yuan points. The first way can be done by sedating the yuan point (kid 3) of the kidney meridian and tonifying the luo point (UB 58) of the bladder meridian. The second way can be done by sedating the luo point (kid 4) of the kidney meridian and tonifying the yuan point (UB 64) of the bladder meridian. Actually, there is nothing that will confuse the reader. In both ways, we sedated the kidney and tonified the bladder. The Yin energy in the kidney meridian changed polarity and was pushed to the bladder meridian as Yang energy. Therefore, Yin decreased and Yang increased. We compared Yin Yang pair channels to fountains of hot and cold water. This polarity change is normal in energy transitions from hot water fountain to cold water fountain or from cold water fountain to hot water fountain. Since the energy appearances of yin yang pair organs are similar to each other, there is no polarity change in deep energy transitions between them (Figure 111).

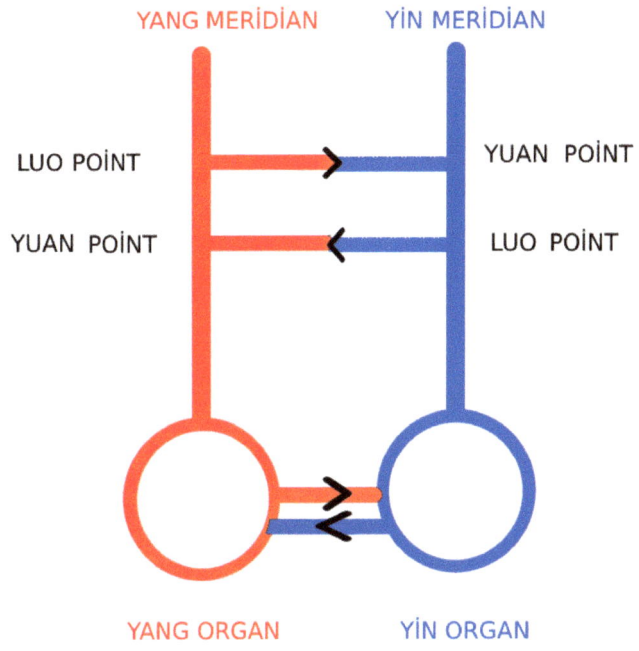

Figure 111: Energy transitions between sister organ and meridian

EXAMPLE CASE 2 (HEARING LOSS):

The examination of the patient, whose hearing loss had gradually started in the ears for five years, revealed that he could not hear bilateral whispers and his rinne test was negative bilaterally. After audiological examination, the patient was diagnosed with otosclerosis. In the tongue examination, a cleft was observed in the tongue corpus from posterior to anterior, the tongue fur was partially thick and yellow in color, and the tongue tip was hyperemic. Although there were no tooth marks, the tongue body was swollen (Figure 112). The pulse was felt superficially and partially thickly in the posterior and middle positions on the right side. Felt slippery in the right center.

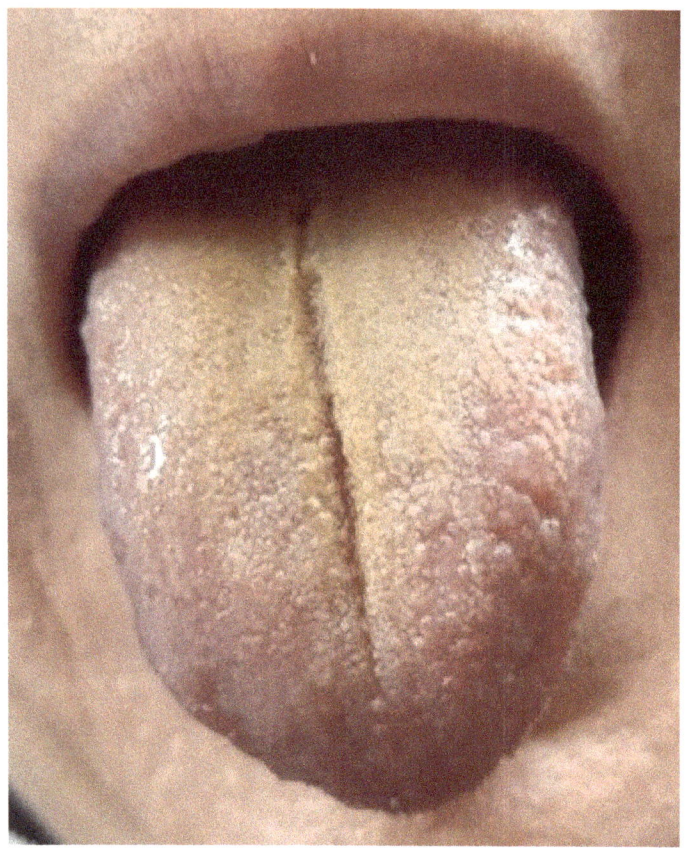

Figure 112: Tongue image

Since the patient's complaint when he came to us was hearing loss, we will first have to turn to the kidney pool as the faulty pool. In the tongue examination, there is a cleft in the tongue corpus from posterior to anterior, indicating that the patient also has stomach and heart Yin deficiency, and that the defective target pool should not only be the kidney. Yellow color of the tongue fur, hyperemic tongue tip and presence of a cleft indicate that the pool is hot. In Yin deficiencies, the tongue corpus is generally thin. This tongue corpus is not thin-looking. At the same time, although there is stomach Yin deficiency, there is no loss of tongue fur. On the contrary, there is some thickening and yellowing. Apparently, in this case, there is phlegm accumulation secondary to stomach Yin deficiency. In other words, the patient has both deficiency and excess. In this case, there are three pools in our target and these pools are hot (Figure 113).

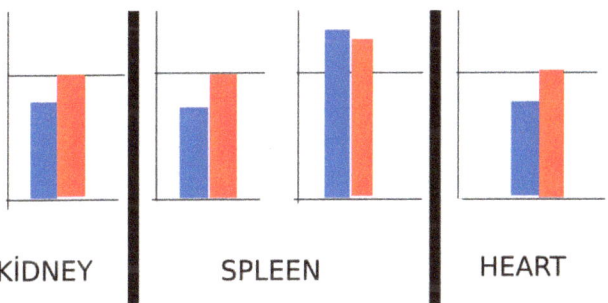

Figure 113: Possible Yin Yang diagrams of target pools

In the Yin Yang diagrams I drew for the target pools, I drew Yang normally, but keep in mind that Yang may also be partially low in chronic cases. I drew it this way because I felt the patient's pulse being somewhat tense.

In light of these findings, it will be sufficient to just turn on the cold water fountain in the kidney and heart pool. Since there is both deficiency and excess in the spleen, pulse examination will guide us on what to do. If the patient had a weak pulse, I would restore the functions of the spleen through tonification and wait for the phlegm to disappear over time. Since I perceived a slippery pulse, I preferred to relieve the phlegm by sedating it. The tonification point (Kid 7) can be used to turn on the cold water fountain of the kidney, the element point with a tonifying maneuver (Kid 10), or the grandmother point of the bladder (UB 40). The tonification point (He 9), the element point (He 8) with a tonifying maneuver, or the grandmother point of the small intestine (SI 2) can be used to turn on the cold water fountain of the heart. It is not necessary to open all three of these points. I usually use two in practice. I tried to solve the phlegm by sedating the Sp 9 and St 40 points. After the third session, noise began to occur in the patient's ears. This sound was in the form of a rustling sound and was a sound that had not existed before. This sound continued to decrease until the ninth or tenth session, and then it passed. The patient's hearing improved greatly.

I usually add a local point to the treatment in every patient with hearing loss or tinnitus in the ear. I needle the points GB 2, SI 19, Sj 21, listed in front of the tragus, with a single needle in an oblique manner and in an open mouth position. I usually add Sj 17 and GB 20 points to these.

Acupuncture is such a beautiful form of treatment that if you do the right things, the results you get can often surprise you. According to Western Medicine, this patient has no choice but to undergo surgery or use a device. The patient is a patient who comes to me from time to time for different reasons. No regression was observed in the hearing of the patient, who was followed for approximately five years.

EXAMPLE CASE 3 (ACCHILLES TENDENITIS):

The patient, who has been describing severe pain on the heel of his left foot for 2-3 months while walking on the road or going up and down the stairs, was relieved by applying cold or resting. In the physical examination of the patient, who was diagnosed with Achilles tendinitis, the right side proximal pulse was felt as thin and tense as a wire. On tongue examination, the tongue body was observed to be dry. Apart from this, no pathological image was detected. What should our treatment plan be like for the patient?

Since there is a kidney meridian on one side of the heel and a bladder meridian on the other, heel-related disorders are treated through the water element. If the pain occurs with movement and is relieved with rest and cold application, this indicates that the pool is hot. Tongue and pulse findings also confirm this. Since the case is in the subacute stage, we expect a Yin Yang diagram in which Yang increases and Yin decreases in the patient (Figure 114).

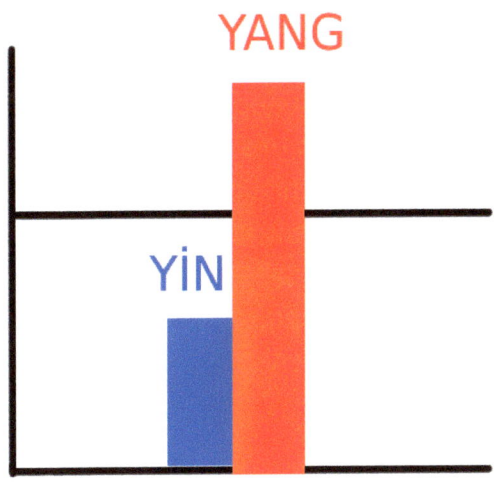

Figure 114: Yang hyperactivity due to Yin deficiency

In this case, what we need to do for the patient is to turn down the hot water fountain and turn on the cold water fountain. To turn on the cold water fountain, the tonification point of the kidney meridian (kid 7), the element point with a tonifying maneuver (kid 10) or the grandmother point of the bladder meridian (UB 40) can be used. The son point (UB 65) or grandson point (UB 60) of the bladder meridian can be used to turn off the hot water fountain. UB 60 point is also more preferred as it is a local point. What would your answer be if I asked you if we could use Kid 3 point as a local point in this patient? Since Kid 3 point is the grandmother point of the kidney meridian, it increases Yang. This is not something we want. This point can be used with a heat-relieving sedation maneuver. In this maneuver, the needle is entered at one level while pushing it down, and it is pulled at three different levels when pulling it up (Figure 115). Also, In cases of lateral epicondylitis, the needle can be used in this way when we use the LI 11 point as a local point.

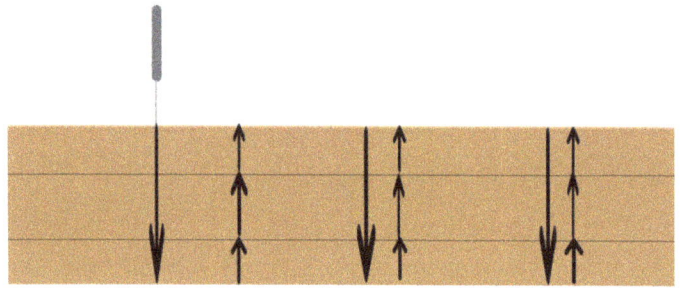

Figure 115: Heat release maneuver

Since tendons are associated with the tree element, it would be appropriate to add the nene point (GB 34) to the treatment via the gallbladder meridian. This point is also one of the eight effective points and is the effective point of the tendons.

EXAMPLE CASE 4 (COMMON JOINT PAIN):

The patient had widespread joint pain for years and this pain was exacerbated in cold and humid weather. The patient experienced stiffness for a while when he woke up in the morning, and his pain decreased throughout the day. The patient, who said that his feet were especially cold, that he urinated frequently, and that his urine was usually copious and light colored every time he came out, did not drink water because he was afraid of being unable to hold his urine in unexpected places if he was going to go out of the house. The tongue body was observed to be wide and pale, and the tongue fur was partially thick and white. The pulse was felt weak, deep and wide on the right side posterior. What should our treatment plan be like for the patient?

In common joint pains that do not describe a specific meridian, our target pool should be kidney. If the patient's pain is aggravated in cold and damp weather, it indicates that the pool is cold. Patients with defficient kidney yang often suffer from the inability to warm their feet. These patients usually wear layers of socks even in summer. The patient's pulse and tongue findings also support that the defective pool is cold. The pulse finding and the fact that the complaint has been going on for years supports that the case is a case of defficiency. In the light of these findings, the Yin Yang diagram we expect in the patient is as follows (Figure 116).

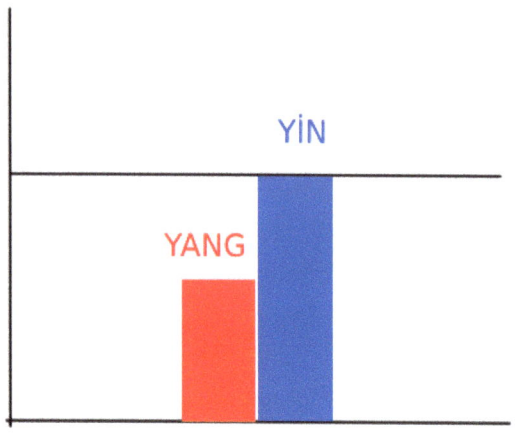

Figure 116: Empty cold

What we need to do for the patient is to turn on the hot water fountain. For this purpose, the tonification point of the bladder meridian (UB 67), the element point with the tonifying maneuver (UB 66), and the grandmother point of the kidney meridian (Kid 3) are useful points. It would also be good to apply moxa to Kid 1 point.

Morning stiffness is evidence of moisture accumulation in the body. For this purpose, the St 40 point can be used with a tonifying maneuver. In this case, Sp 9 (Lasix point) is not considered as it will increase the Yin load of the kidney.

EXAMPLE CASE 5 (TINNITUS):

The patient started experiencing ringing in his left ear approximately 5-6 years ago after being exposed to a loud sound, and this complaint increased when he was overtired, sleep deprived, and during periods of intense stress. On tongue examination, the tongue body was observed to be partially hyperemic and dry, and the tongue rust was yellow (Figure 117). The pulse was felt as thin, superficial and partially tense in the proximal position on the right side. What should our treatment plan be like for the patient?

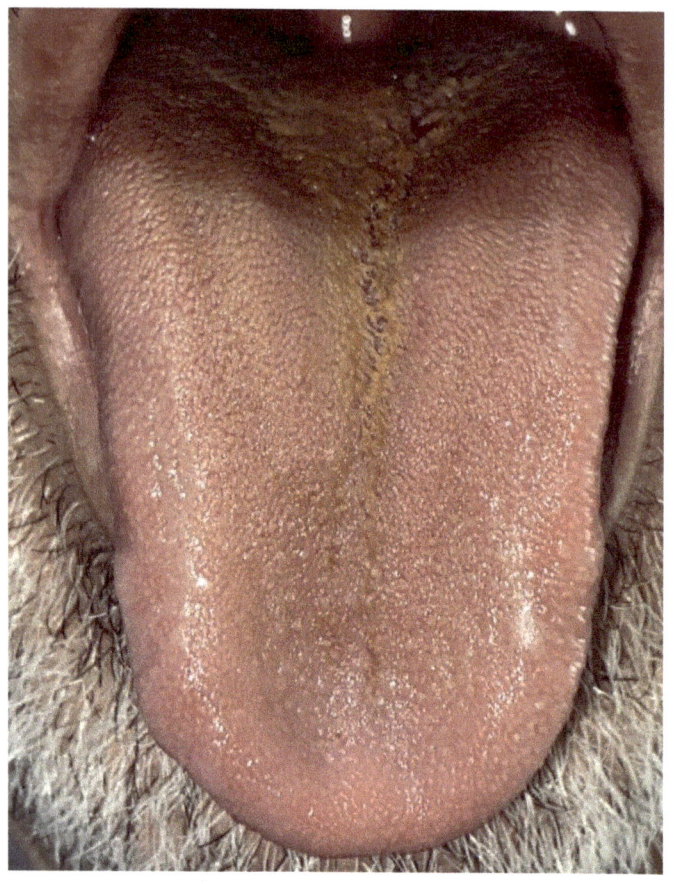

Figure 117: Tongue image

Since the ear is the sensory organ associated with the water element, we considered the kidney and bladder as the defective pool. The patient's tongue is partially dry and hyperemic, the pulse is superficial and partially tense, indicating that the pool is hot. The prolonged duration of the complaint and the fine pulse are evidence of a case of insufficiency. In the light of these findings, the Yin Yang diagram we expect in the patient is as follows (Figure 118).

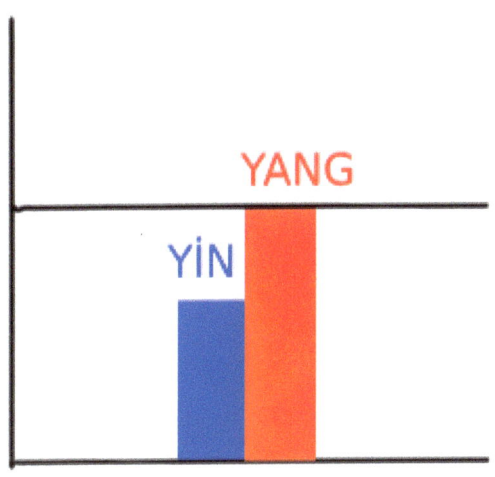

Figure 118: Empty hot

In this case, the only thing we need to do in the patient is to open the cold water tap. For this purpose, the tonification point of the renal meridian (Kid 7), the element point with tonifying maneuver (Kid 10) or the nene point of the bladder (UB 40) were used. As local points, GB 2, SI 19 and Sj 21 points were pricked obliquely with a single needle. GB 20 and Sj 17 points were also used as local points. Two sessions per week were performed for a total of 10 sessions. After the treatment, the complaint was relieved to a great extent.

If I had taken this patient's pulse as weak instead of slightly tense, I would have thought that the Yin Yang diagram was as shown in the figure below (Figure 119).

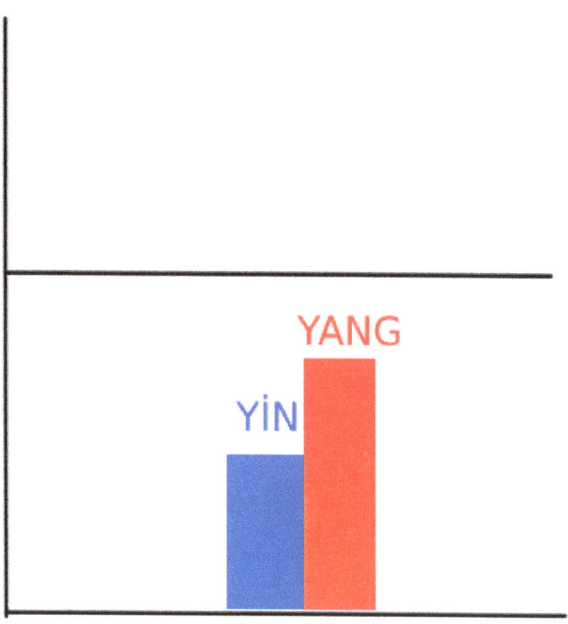

Figure 119: Empty hot

In this case, I would add a hot water fountain, such as Kid 3, to the three cold water fountains I mentioned above.

I assume that the sample cases related to the water element are sufficient to understand the subject. Thus, we have finished the five shu points of all elements and examples of how they are used in the clinic. In the book, I tried to present the approach to diseases in a very systematic way. If you have learned acupuncture in the way I have described, if you have grasped the logic of the approach to diseases, you can do the work of rebalancing the disturbed Yin Yang balance through different points in treatment. But my advice to you is to use the five shu points first. Over time, when you include other points in your applications on the same logic, your treatment success rate will increase day by day. Do not neglect tongue and pulse examination in every patient, even if you do not understand them. To reach the last rung of the ladder, you must first step on the first rung. Perfection and faultlessness are reserved for Allah. No matter how much attention I pay, there will be mistakes and errors in the book. If the deficiencies are communicated to me, we will try to correct them. Good health to you.

RESOURCES

- Radha Thambirajah, Energetics in Acupuncture, Five Element Acupuncture, Second Edition 2008
- Radha Thambirajah, Cosmetic Acupuncture, A traditional Chinese Medicine Approach to Cosmetic and Dermatological Problems, 2009
- Giovanni Maciocia, The Foundations of Chinese Medicine, third edition, 2015
- Giovanni Maciocia, The Practice of Chinese Medicine, The Treatment of Diseases with Acupuncture and Chinese Herbs, Second Edition, 2008
- Giovanni Macciocia, Tongue Diagnosis in Chinese Medicine, Revised Edition, Fifth Printing, 2000
- Hans-Urlich Hecker, Angelika Steveling, Elmar T. Peuker, Joerg Kastner, Practice of Acupuncture, Point location-Tecniques- Treatment Options
- Claudia Focks, Atlas of Acupuncture, Second Edition 2006
- Stux, Berman, Pomeranz, Basic of Acupuncture, 5 th Edition, 2003
- Chen Jirui, Nissi Wang, Acupuncture Case Histories from China, 1988

- Evidence-Based Complementary and Alternative Medicine Volume 2015, Article ID 361974, 17 pages
- Open Access Library Journal > Vol.4 No.12, December 2017, Five Parifhases Music Therapy (FPMT) in Chinese Medicine: Fundamentals and Application, Hui Zhang, Han Lai
- The Five Elements And Other Essential Rules In Acupuncture Treatment, By Ulrich Wilhelm Lippelt
- Classical chinese medicine, liu lihong
- Martin Wang, More Than Acupuncture: Questions and Answers about Chinese Medicine, First edition 2018
- Introduction to Formulae of Traditional Chinese Medicine, Jin Yang, Huang Huang, Li-jiang Zhu, 2005

www.ingramcontent.com/pod-product-compliance
Lightning Source LLC
LaVergne TN
LVHW050130080526
838202LV00061B/6459